Healing Cancer
From Inside Out

A Practical Guide to Healing Cancer
with
The RAVE Diet & Lifestyle

by
Mike Anderson

Published by
www.RaveDiet.com

International Standard Book Number (ISBN)
978-0-9726590-5-5

First Edition: April 2009

Printed in the United States of America

To my father.

Acknowledgments

Many people contributed to the making of this book and the film of the same title. I would like to thank the following individuals who volunteered their time and talented efforts to make both possible.

Marion Albert
Rosemary Byrne
T. Colin Campbell, Ph.D.
Brian Clement, Ph.D.
Brenda Cobb
Mirea Ellis
Charlotte Gerson
John Hoffman
Matt Lederman, M.D.
Thomas Lodi, M.D.
John A. McDougall, M.D.
Pam Navarro
Mariana Pina-Bergtold

Disclaimer

If you have any medical condition, you should change your diet only under the care of a physician. Neither the author nor any advisors for this book make any representation or warranty of any kind whatsoever regarding the appropriateness of the advice contained herein for any individual. The information presented is not medical advice and is not given as medical advice. If you need a physician to work with you, please visit the web site at www.RaveDiet.com.

Table of Contents

Introduction

"During the past fifty years scientists experimenting with thousands of animals have found 700 ways of causing cancer. But they have not discovered one way of curing the disease." – J. F. Brailsford, M.D.

The purpose of this book is to support the film of the same name, *Healing Cancer From Inside Out.* If you haven't seen the film, you should pick up a copy[1] because it contains vital information not found here. This book focuses on providing the details for supporting cancer patients with nutrition and essentially picks up where the film leaves off. The exception is Part I, where I provide a detailed explanation of how ineffective – and harmful – current conventional treatments are to the cancer patient.

This book is both a summary and interpretation of what I've discovered over the years about healing cancer with diet. It is based on the best scientific and practitioner knowledge to date. What I hope is that the material presented in this book will enable those with cancer to make their own treatment decisions based on *all* the facts.

I am neither for nor against conventional treatments of cancer. Nor am I for or against alternative treatments of cancer. What I am for is *any* treatment that truly works, particularly those that work in the long run and keep cancer away for good.

As made clear in the film, the difference between cancer prevention and reversal is one of degree, not kind. Natural cancer reversals occur all the time. At this moment, there are millions of people with cancers growing in their bodies and they don't have a clue. In fact, the average American gets half a dozen serious bouts of cancer during his or her lifetime without even knowing it![2] This means there are millions of people who have healed their cancers on their own – including you. It also means that, overall, there are many more natural cancer reversals than there are diagnosed and treated cancer cases.

Obviously, the more a cancer has progressed, the more difficult it will be to reverse. In other words, the sooner you adopt a true cancer-fighting diet, the better your chances of reversing the cancer and never having it return. Dietary reversals have occurred in all stages of cancer, including patients who were given only a few months to live, so you should never give up hope or stop fighting this disease.

The diet outlined in this book is strict, as it has to be. The closer you adhere to it, the more effective it will be. The basic guidelines are taken from the book, *The Rave Diet & Lifestyle*, which I also authored. The book you're reading now contains guidelines specifically tailored to fight the disease, as well as much

---

[1] Healing Cancer From Inside Out is available at www.RaveDiet.com.
[2] Patrick Quillin, Ph.D., Beating Cancer with Nutrition, p. 10.

more information about cancer. Once the cancer is under control, you can return to a more relaxed diet with wider food choices, such as that outlined in the *Rave Diet & Lifestyle*.

Dr. Bernie Siegel has said that when given a choice between a change in lifestyle and undergoing surgery, eight out of ten patients will say, "operate."[3] The two people out of ten who choose lifestyle changes, he calls "extraordinary" because they have chosen a different path – one that addresses the cause of the problem instead of having the doctor treat a symptom. Because you are reading this book, you should consider yourself an extraordinary individual because you have the courage to walk a path that is not well-trodden. That path is full of long-term successes which have rid the body of cancer not just for a few years, but a lifetime. I want to personally congratulate you for your decision. As you read the book and adopt the diet, you will find that you are not alone and have many resources to support you.

There is a story about a professor of medicine who would always make jokes about heart attacks to his medical students and the jokes would always elicit laughter. One day, he thought he would augment his heart disease jokes with some about cancer. But when he told the jokes, no one laughed. Of course, the reason no one laughed is because we have no effective treatments for cancer. Cancer is seen, by most, for what it is today with conventional treatments: a death sentence for all but a very few. And, yet, it doesn't have to be.

We can make jokes about heart disease despite the fact that it kills as many people as cancer. And cardiovascular disease, of which heart disease is a subset, kills over *twice* as many people as cancer does. This is not to say that any disease is a laughing matter, but to point out that we have a very different attitude about cancer than we have about other diseases. Much of that attitude stems from the fact that conventional medicine has no effective treatments and, as a result, doctors are all too often giving patients death sentences. They have tried their ineffective treatments, the patient is told there are *no alternatives* and therefore the patient has only "x" number of months to live.

Sentencing a patient to death is the worst thing a doctor can do. The doctor is giving the patient a nocebo – the opposite of a placebo – which is, in effect, a kind of hex, whose underlying message to the patient is to die. So what does the patient do? He goes home, grapples with his fate and dies right on schedule. The doctor expects the patient will die and the patient follows the doctor's expectations right to his grave. The doctor's prophecy becomes self-fulfilling due to the blind faith patients have in modern medicine.

When patients are told there is no alternative but death, that's criminal because there *are* alternatives, even with late stage cancers. Unfortunately, the medical culture and legal system limit treatment options to the worst therapies ever to

---

[3] Bernie S. Siegel, M.D., Love, Medicine & Miracles.

visit the human body. Doctors are ignorant of any treatment beyond drugs, radiation and surgery. Hope is dead and so, too, will be the patient.

"Drugs tend to worsen whatever they're supposed to cure, which sets up a vicious circle." – Dean Black, M.D.

A common occurrence is what I call the "Cancer Cycle." A person is diagnosed with cancer, treatments are applied, the body is devastated, but the patient is "cured." A few years later, the cancer returns. More treatment is applied, the body is further devastated, and the cancer is once again "cured." A few years later, the cancer returns yet again. At this point, either further treatment kills them or the side effects do.

In fact, the "Cancer Cycle" is so common it's been estimated it occurs, in varying degrees, with over 90 percent of all cases where treatments are rendered.[4]

Why? Because conventional medicine only treats the symptoms of cancer (e.g., a tumor) and does not address what caused the cancer in the first place. Since the dose of radiation or chemo required to kill *all* cancer cells would also kill the patient, you still have malignant cancer cells in your body even after you have been "cured," they're just hiding under the radar. Normally, your body could deal with this, but the treatments have devastated your immune system and set the stage for the return of a serious cancer. This is the fundamental problem with conventional treatments: They damage the body so much that it is incapable of defending itself against cancer. And this is what sets up the Cancer Cycle.

Adding injury to insult, radiological and chemo treatments actually increase the likelihood that cancer will develop in other parts of the body[5] because both of these treatments are active carcinogens! Don't you think it's strange that one of the possible side effects of our cancer treatments is cancer itself?

Women who received radiation treatment and survived early Hodgkin's cancers, for example, were 75 times more likely to develop breast cancer by age 45![6] As Dr. Samuel S. Epstein has said, "Chemotherapy and radiation can increase the risk of developing a second cancer by up to 100 times."[7]

---

[4] You will hear lower figures, but these refer to a recurrence of a specific *type* of cancer, e.g., breast cancer. We are talking about a recurrence of cancer, regardless of the type. This means the body is still making cancer and it simply shows up as a different type of cancer, in a different area of the body. See *Part 2* for more on this.

[5] Chemotherapy releases an abundance of oxidants, which are highly reactive oxygen molecules that support the life of cancer. This not only makes the conditions within the body hospitable to the cancer, but toxic to the immune system, thus further encouraging the life of the disease. Instead of strengthening the immune system, chemo devastates it.

[6] Breast Cancer and Other Second Neoplasms after Childhood Hodgkin's Disease, S. Bhatia, et al., NEJM, 1996, 334:745-51.

[7] Samuel S. Epstein, M.D., Congressional Record, Sept. 9, 1987

Chemotherapy is advertised as somewhat effective against a very small number of cancers: Hodgkin's disease, acute lymphocytic leukemia, testicular cancer and choriocarcinoma. When you look at its long-term effectiveness, however, the value of the treatment diminishes over time.

A study of over 10,000 patients with Hodgkin's, who were treated with chemo, showed they were 14 times more likely to develop leukemia and six times more likely to develop cancers of the bones, joints and soft tissues than those patients who did not undergo chemotherapy.[8] Children who were "successfully" treated for Hodgkin's are 18 times more likely to later develop secondary malignant tumors; the risk of leukemia increases markedly just four years after the treatment has ended; and the risk of developing solid tumors approaches 30 percent after 30 years.[9]

With childhood cancers, 73 percent of patients will develop a chronic illness within 30 years and 42 percent will develop a severe, disabling, life-threatening or fatal condition, including heart disease, lung scarring, strokes and second cancers.[10] Blindness, deafness, infertility, early menopause, neurocognitive defects, depression, anxiety and moderate to extreme physical pain are also common side effects. Many have bones more osteoporotic in their 20s than people in their 70s. And no one has ever seen a childhood survivor make it to 70 years of age. It's no wonder that survivors of such treatments are advised to find jobs at big companies with good medical insurance!

A study of women who survived ovarian cancer following chemo treatments showed a 100-fold greater incidence of leukemia over those who did not receive chemotherapy. In some studies, when chemo and radiation were combined, the incidence of secondary tumors was 25 times the expected rate.[11]

In other words, the Cancer Cycle can have a very long and painful time frame because the treatment itself often causes later death from secondary cancers and other treatment-related diseases. And along the way, the treatment will enter the books as a success because the patient survived for just five years. Someone who

---

[8] NCI Journal 87:10.

[9] NEJM, March 21, 1996.

[10] Philip M. Rosoff, M.D. The Two-Edged Sword of Curing Childhood Cancer. Volume 355:1522-1523, No. 15.

[11] Discussed in Seeds of Destruction: The Science Report on Cancer Research, Thomas A. Maugh and Jean L. Marx. On a related topic, one reason why cancers seem to return with such a vengeance after chemo treatments is that cancer cells resist the drug by replicating even harder and faster than before the chemo (they are in a survival mode, after all). Chemo drugs are lethal so cancer cells are stimulated to survive in any way they can, which results in faster growth. In the presence of any lethal drug, they resist and the more they resist, the stronger they get. This is simply an adaptation by cancer cells to stay alive. The chemo provokes this adaptation and the rapid cancer growth can quickly overwhelm a patient. Of course, the chemo knocks down the immune system and the cancer regains its powers and starts growing long before the immune system is strong enough to combat the illness.

dies of pneumonia, because his or her immune system was destroyed by chemotherapy, for example, is generally not counted as a "cancer" death. Likewise, someone whose liver is destroyed by chemo, and dies of liver disease, is also not counted as a cancer death. Cancer mortality as a result of treatment is grossly *understated* because the cause of death is taken from a death certificate. The direct cause of death may have been liver failure, but the liver failure was caused by the treatment. Because of the way deaths are recorded, it makes "cure" rates look far better than they actually are.[12] In fact, it's been said that if you add up treatment-related deaths, conventional cancer treatments have done far more harm than good.

Because you are reading this, you no doubt have cancer, or know someone who does. With such a serious disease, not everyone gets well, no matter what program they follow. That's the nature of life and this disease. But if you play the odds and follow a strict program of diet and lifestyle changes, your chances of beating cancer will skyrocket, compared to if you did not follow these guidelines.

When you heal the body nutritionally, you heal the entire body – the heart, liver, spleen, colon and every single cell in your body. In contrast, our current medical model uses powerful poisons to rearrange body chemistry in order to suppress *symptoms* of the disease. It also cuts out or surgically alters organs that are causing problems, instead of healing those organs. The beauty about diet and lifestyle changes is that you don't have to know a thing about cancer to reverse it. You just have to know a thing or two about what you put into your mouth and how to live your life. The purpose of this book is to tell you a thing or two about how to do both.

If you are diagnosed with cancer, fear will undoubtedly cloud your judgment, which can lead you down that slippery slope of hasty, regrettable decisions. Even though the cancer has taken years, if not decades to develop, the doctors will tell you that you must have chemo and/or radiation and/or surgery *immediately*! They will also use scare tactics to try to force you into treatment ("You will *die* if you don't have treatment" is the usual phrase). Here is what I would suggest:

1) Read the rest of this book.
2) Start the diet. Don't wait. It doesn't hurt and will only help. The side effects are all beneficial.

---

[12] Cancer registries, such as the NCI's SEER database, rely solely on information provided by death certificates. And, yet, cause of death is often recorded as something else, when in fact the underlying cause is advanced metastasized cancer. Cancer mortality is also underestimated due to the steady decline in the number of autopsies done on patients who die in hospitals. In the US, the autopsy rate has plummeted from around 45 per cent several decades ago to only around 11 per cent today. Some hospitals now perform autopsies on fewer than 5 per cent of patients who die there.

3) Get a second opinion, a second diagnosis. Cancer diagnoses can be problematic. See the chapter on early screening for an example with mammograms.
4) Get your markers re-checked after a few months. If you've found you're making progress, that you're turning the tide, keep on the diet and stay the course.
5) If you are not making progress, then you have more decisions to make. I would advise that you get professional help from a clinic which has experience reversing cancers using natural means, as you may be in need of specialized treatments. For clinic references, see www.RaveDiet.com.

If you have cancer and accept standard treatments, you may get some relief in the short-term, but statistically, you have set yourself up for the Cancer Cycle. Those few people who have escaped the Cycle were those who took charge of their health and changed their diets and lifestyles.[13] If you are a survivor of conventional treatments, it is just as important for you to adopt the dietary guidelines in this book in order to escape the Cycle.[14]

There are literally hundreds of alternative cancer treatments out there, which rely on one supplement, or another, or one specialized type of treatment or another. (See *Part 3 – Supplementation.*) Instead of focusing on supplementation, this book discusses nutrition because nutrition is the foundation for reversing cancer, regardless of supplementation. Nutrition can reverse cancer by itself. It can also reverse cancer in conjunction with supplements or specialized treatments. But supplements and specialized treatments cannot reverse cancers on their own, particularly in the long run. In other words, if you are serious about reversing cancer, you should be serious about changing your diet and lifestyle because that is what will keep cancer out of your body for good.

Should you follow this diet if you are undergoing conventional treatments?

The short answer is yes, you should adopt this diet, even when undergoing conventional treatments.

Will it interfere with my treatment?

Absolutely not!

There has recently been a lot of press about antioxidants interfering with radiation treatments because of a study. There are two important points about that study which need to be clarified. First, a subsequent analysis (after the headlines)

---

[13] Horii R, Akiyama F, Kasumi F, Koike M, Sakamoto G. Spontaneous "healing" of breast cancer. Breast Cancer. 2005;12(2):140-4; Larsen SU, Rose C. Spontaneous remission of breast cancer. A literature review. Ugeskr Laeger. 1999 Jun 28;161(26): 4001-4; Lifestyle Changes and the 'Spontaneous' Regression of Cancer…, Foster, H, Inter. Jnl Biosocial Research, 10(1), 1988, pp. 17-33; Healing Cancer From Inside Out (film), Mike Anderson.
[14] Jaiswal McEligot A, Largent J, Ziogas A, Peel D, Anton-Culver H. Dietary fat, fiber, vegetable, and micronutrients are associated with overall survival in postmenopausal women diagnosed with breastcancer. Nutr Cancer. 2006;55(2):132-40.

showed that the danger of antioxidants was limited to a sub-population, specifically those who continued to smoke cigarettes during radiation treatment.[15] Secondly – and more important – patients were taking *synthetic* antioxidant supplements, not the natural antioxidants that you get from eating whole foods. Antioxidants from natural, whole foods will *never* interfere will any treatment.

In another study, *synthetic* beta-carotene *supplements* increased the risk for lung cancer in heavy smokers.[16] Along the same lines, a recent study showed that a combination of vitamins E, C and selenium *supplements* were useless for combating prostate cancer.[17] I could not agree more with these studies. Synthetic supplements, on their own, will never make a dent against cancer.

When you get your antioxidants, vitamins, minerals and other micronutrients from natural, whole foods, not only will there never be a problem, but they are far more powerful than supplements. Synthetic (man-made) supplements are not only weaklings against the powerhouse of natural foods, but taking them on a long-term basis can very often lead to diseases. (See *Part 3 – Supplementation.*)

Will dietary treatment actually work when undergoing conventional treatments?

They will be far less successful than if you had no conventional therapy at all. Why? Because the purpose of dietary treatments is to rebuild the body's defenses, particularly the immune system, and conventional treatments do the opposite – they devastate the immune system, as well as every organ and cell in the body. It's as if nutritional therapy were trying to build a fence to keep cancer out, while conventional therapy tears it down. In other words, dietary treatment can help during conventional treatments, but it is an uphill battle. It takes years for the immune system to recover from chemotherapy. Dietary treatments can help it recover sooner, but the treatments themselves make this much more difficult. Without question, you will improve your chances of long-term survival after treatment by following the diet.

The overwhelming fear of cancer should tell you more than anything else that after decades of research and over a trillion dollars of aimless spending, our current medical model does not cure cancer. In fact, as will become apparent, this model doesn't have a chance at *ever* finding a cure. It is simply the wrong approach to the disease.

---

[15] Meyer F, Bairati I, Fortin A, et al. Interaction between antioxidant vitamin supplementation and cigarette smoking during radiation therapy in relation to long-term effects on recurrence and mortality: A randomized trial among head and neck cancer patients. Int J Cancer. 2007 Dec 4;122(7):1679-168.
[16] Goodman GE, et al. The Beta-Carotene and Retinol Efficacy Trial: incidence of lung cancer and cardiovascular disease mortality during 6-year follow-up after stopping beta-carotene and retinol supplements. J Natl Cancer Inst. 2004 Dec 1;96(23):1729-31.
[17] The home page for this study can be found here: www.crab.org/select/. Vitamin C was added in a follow-up study.

Because you are reading this book, it means you are among the 15 to 20 percent of people who are "rule breakers," who think on their own and are capable of making their own decisions about their health and treatment.[18] The majority of patients are like actors auditioning for a part – they perform to satisfy the physician and will do whatever he or she decides. The patient is merely a passive participant and not required to do anything about their illness, except pay the bills and obediently follow the instructions of the doctor.

At the other end of the spectrum are those patients who actually wish to die – either consciously or subconsciously – and welcome the diagnosis as a way to escape their problems.[19]

The rule breakers are active participants in their health care, who will not play the victim and will do things on their own. That is what you must be if you are to follow this program.

I wish I had the information in this book when my father was struck with cancer. He died and there was nothing I, nor he, could do – simply because we knew of no alternative. It is my sincere hope this material will help with your situation.

This book is about keeping you alive as long as possible. Conventional medicine is about allowing you to die as long as possible. This book is about raising your quality of life. Conventional medicine is about using treatments that degrade and debase your life. This book is about allowing you to squeeze as much life out of every day that you possibly can. Conventional medicine is about making you feel like a prisoner on death row, praying for a pardon. Ultimately, this book is about helping you make an escape from that prison so you can become a free person, on your own, once again.

---

[18] For more on this, see Bernie S. Siegel, M.D., Love, Medicine & Miracles, p. 22.
[19] Ibid, p. 22-23.

PART 1 – The Failure of Conventional Treatments

Show Me the Money

"The American public is being sold a nasty bill of goods." – Dr. James Watson, Nobel Prize Winner while serving on the National Cancer Advisory Board, 1975

"For most of today's common solid cancers, the ones that cause 90% of the cancer deaths each year, chemotherapy has never proven to do any good at all." – Urich Abel, M.D., University of Heidelberg, 1990

"Evidence has steadily accrued that [cancer therapy] is essentially a failure." – N.J. Temple, M.D., Journal of the Royal Society of Medicine, 1991

"We have given it our best effort for decades: billions of dollars of support, the best scientific talent available. It hasn't paid off." – John C. Bailar, M.D., Harvard University, 1997

"Survival gains for the more common forms of cancer are measured in additional months of life, not years...." – Fortune Magazine, 2004

"The National Cancer Institute and the American Cancer Society have misled and confused the public and Congress by repeated false claims that we are winning the war against cancer – claims made to create public and Congressional support for massive increases in budgetary appropriations." – Samuel S. Epstein, M.D.

Ultimately, I'm a pragmatist. Show me something that works and I'll use it. If it doesn't work, I won't use it. In all but a very few cases, conventional cancer treatments simply do not work. Due to clever number manipulation, however, the cancer industry has made it appear as if treatments for the vast majority of cancers *do* work. Unfortunately, they don't. And this sad fact has been known since the war on cancer began.

One of the best large-scale studies on the effectiveness of chemotherapy treatments – the main weapon in the cancer war – was published in 2004. This study was not conducted by some wild-eyed, angry scientist, but two highly respected oncologists from Australia. They simply looked at the results of every randomized, controlled clinical trial performed in the U.S. between 1990 and 2004, which reported a statistically significant increase in five-year survival due to the use of chemotherapy. That is, they looked at the number of cancer patients who survived more than five years following diagnosis and treatment. Here are the results:[1]

Cancer	Percent 5-Year Survival
Bladder	00.0
Kidney	00.0
Melanoma	00.0
Multiple myeloma	00.0
Pancreas	00.0
Prostate	00.0
Soft tissue sarcoma	00.0
Unknown primary site	00.0
Uterus	00.0
Stomach	00.7
Colon	01.0
Breast	01.4
Head and Neck	01.9
Lung	02.0
Rectum	03.4
Brain	03.7
Esophagus	04.9
Ovary	08.9
Non-Hodgkin's lymphoma	10.5
Cervix	12.0
Testis	37.7
Hodgkin's disease	40.3
Overall 5-Year Survival Rate	**2.1**

There are several interesting things to note about this study. First, not a single major newspaper or other media outlet covered it in the US. Now, this is a study covering chemotherapy treatments over a 14-year time span by two respected

---

[1] Clinical Oncology (2004) 16: 549-560. It should be noted the authors also studied treatments in Australia and the results were virtually identical to those in the US. This should come as no surprise. Other studies over the years have come to the same conclusion. In 1985, Scientific American published a landmark study which revealed chemo was only effective in *two to three percent* of all cancer cases. (John Cairns, The Treatment of Diseases and the War Against Cancer, Scientific American, Vol. 253, No. 5.) In 1990, a renowned biostatistics expert reviewed chemotherapy-treated cancer patients and concluded that chemo can help only *three percent* of patients with epithelial cancers, such as breast, prostate, colon and lung cancers. See Abel Urich, Chemotherapy of Advanced Epithelial Cancer: A Critical Survey, Hippokrates Verlag Stuttgart, 1990.

oncologists and the results contradict everything that has been spoon-fed to the press. One would think the public would be interested in knowing just how ineffective chemo really is, particularly since their tax dollars are plowed into research that supports the pharmaceutical companies making these drugs. The media obviously thought it was not newsworthy, despite the fact that they regularly report "good news" on the cancer front.

This study had very little coverage even in the authors' native Australia.[2] On a radio show,[3] the host brought in one of the top oncologists in Australia, Dr. Michael Boyer, Head of Medical Oncology at the Sydney Cancer Centre, to comment on the study. While not questioning the validity of the study, his major complaint was that the authors used "absolute" numbers instead of "relative" numbers (more on this below). Dr. Boyer opined that chemo treatments in the "real world" were *much* higher than in clinical trials. Instead of an overall five-year survival rate of just two percent, the five-year survival rate for chemo treatments was probably a whopping five or six percent!

Now, the medical profession generally considers any drug with less than a 30 percent effectiveness to be no better than a placebo.[4] What you have is a top oncologist stating that chemo is effective only five or six percent of the time. Translation: Your chances of surviving more than five years would be better if you took a sugar pill – with a whiskey chaser!

Unfortunately, that's not a bad joke. The few studies that have been done comparing the benefits of conventional treatments versus doing nothing, show that people who did nothing actually lived as long, if not longer, than those who underwent treatments – and obviously had a much higher quality of life![5] (See *The Do Nothing Strategy*.)

You might be asking, if conventional treatments are so ineffective, how can medical professionals sleep at night after putting patients through what, in many cases, are life-threatening treatments. Dr. Michael Boyer himself gives us the answer:

---

[2] Segelov, E. The emperor's new clothes – can chemotherapy survive? Australian Prescriber. 2006; 29 (1):2-3.

[3] The Health Report, Norman Swan, www.abc.net.au/rn/talks/8.30/helthrpt/stories/s1348333.htm

[4] Conventional medicine has always used the placebo effect as an excuse for not validating alternative treatments – that the effectiveness of acupuncture, for example, could be ascribed to the placebo effect. It's duplicitous that they do not apply the same standard to chemo and other cancer treatments which are far less effective than a placebo. To put it bluntly, they approve treatments that are profitable, regardless of the standards they, themselves, have laid down.

[5] JAMA, 1992, 257, p. 2191; Lancet, 1991, August, p. 901; NEJM, 1986, May 27, p. 967; NEJM, 1984, March, p. 737; Cancer, 1981, 47, p. 27; JAMA. 1979;241:489-494; A Report on Cancer, 1969, Hardin Jones.

"...it's not true to say that because you have to [treat] 20 or 25 people to benefit one, it's not true to say that nobody benefits."[6]

In other words, even if only four people out of 100 "benefit" from these treatments, then it's worth it. It's worth subjecting all 100 people to these horrific treatments in order to benefit four.

But two questions arise: 1) what happened to the other 96 people (aside from the fact they had to endure these horrific treatments)? They are obviously in their graves. Can you think of any other profession in the world that would classify such a miserable success rate...as success? 2) How is it possible to claim that four people benefited from a treatment when the benefit is so low that the recovery could easily be attributed to the placebo effect? With such poor results, it's simply a huge leap of faith to say that treatments were responsible for the recovery. Using the medical profession's own standards, a sugar pill would have had better results – and without injuring everyone.

When conventional medicine can talk about a 70 percent rate of effectiveness, then we can believe such treatments may be working. But that gets us into another problematic area. They *do* speak of treatments with a 70 percent (plus) cure rate. How do they get away with this? By manipulating numbers.

When a doctor tells a patient a treatment has a 70 percent cure rate, the patient obviously thinks that 70 people out of 100 will be cured. Wouldn't you? The patient is, in all likelihood, not a statistical researcher and the doctor, in all likelihood, is simply rattling off the numbers given to him by the pharmaceutical or radiological industries.

What the doctor is referring to is the "relative" percentage, which is not at all commonsensical and, in this context, downright deceiving. In fact, some might call it fraud. Here is the dictionary definition of fraud:

"deceit, trickery, sharp practice, or breach of confidence, perpetrated for profit or to gain some unfair or dishonest advantage."

Let's look at this fraud with a simple example. If an oncologist were to say that by giving you chemotherapy treatments, your survival rate would increase from three to six percent (a three percent benefit), you would probably reply, "I'd rather visit a witch doctor!" Well, these are absolute numbers, which are always bad news in the cancer industry. (Absolute numbers were used in the study shown above.) But the oncologist's presentation rarely, if ever, uses absolute numbers. Instead, he refers to numbers provided by the cancer industry, which turns the statistic on its head. Instead of a three percent benefit, he exclaims the exact same treatment has a 100 percent benefit!

How can this be? Easy. If a treatment causes survival rates to increase from three percent to six percent, that represents a 100 percent increase in survival

---

[6] http://www.abc.net.au/rn/talks/8.30/helthrpt/stories/s1348333.htm.

rates! These relative or "rubber" numbers are the numbers used universally throughout the cancer industry to mask the massive failure of conventional treatments. The cancer industry lives, breathes and sleeps these numbers because only these numbers provide big pay days. Relative numbers are, in fact, the lingua franca of the industry and how the industry creates the "good news" that you read in newspapers.

Another example. Say there were 100 people involved in a clinical trial of a new chemotherapy drug. Out of the 100, experts expect two people to get breast cancer. But during the trial, after all 100 people were put on the toxic drug, only one person got breast cancer, meaning the reduction in breast cancer was one person out of 100. Again, this is the *absolute benefit*, 1 in 100, or, one percent.

This is not good news for the drug company because 1 in 100 could easily – and would probably – happen by chance. But, remember, two people were expected to get breast cancer, and only one got it – and 1 divided by 2 equals a 50 percent reduction. Through the magic of number manipulation, this drug can all of a sudden reduce your chances of getting breast cancer by a whopping 50 percent! Quite a sales pitch, eh?

Let's take an example from the real world: Herceptin proponents claim clinical trials show a 46 percent decrease in breast cancer recurrence when the drug was prescribed to late-stage breast cancer patients. This is a *relative* statistic. What's the absolute number? 0.6 percent (less than one percent)! We went from a dishonest 46% decrease (which is what patients are told) to an honest 0.6 percent decrease using the exact same data! Why bother taking the drug? It will surely do more harm than good.

A few years back there were headline articles reporting a 49 percent decrease in the incidence of breast cancer in women who took Tamoxifen for five years. Again, this is a *relative* number. The *absolute* number? 1.5 percent. In all cases, far, far less than what you would expect from a sugar pill.

In 2007, headlines screamed that a new drug, Sorafenib, prolonged survival time for liver cancer patients by a whopping 44 percent! What did that translate into, in absolute numbers: three extra months of living hell with that drug.

We don't necessarily want to bad mouth Herceptin or Tamoxifen or Sorafenib. These are just a few examples. The point is that <u>any current treatment has these kinds of feeble numbers</u>! When you hear someone in the cancer industry citing five-year survival rates above a few percentage points, for all but a small handful of cancers, they are deceiving you. They are using manipulated, *relative* numbers.

In order to understand relative statistics, you have to ask "Relative to what?" In the first simple example, the statistic was relative to the *expectation* that only three people out of 100 would survive for five years without the treatment. In the second example, the statistic was relative to the *expectation* that two people out of 100 would get breast cancer over the course of the clinical trial.

In other words, relative numbers do not stand on their own, as absolute numbers do, but stand on another number. They are *derived* numbers. They are derived from an expectation, an assumption, the results of a previous study, the differences between two different treatment methods, etc. They are used to show a treatment's effectiveness, *relative* to something else.

Say a previous study showed no benefit with a particular treatment. Another study comes along and shows that one person out of 100 benefited from that treatment. Compared to the previous study, in which there was zero benefit, the new study would show a 100% benefit! That benefit, in other words, was *relative* to the old study!

Rubber numbers are, in fact, the bread and butter of the cancer industry and the bedrock foundation for justifying the use of screening techniques and treatments that do not work. They are presented to both patients and Congress in an effort to show that ineffective treatments are effective, when in fact they are not. And they are presented to both parties for only one reason: to get money.

To present such warped numbers to patients (or Congress), who have no idea what relative numbers are – much less what they are relative to – amounts to fraud in my opinion. I've had conversations with oncologists who didn't even know the difference between relative and absolute numbers. They just read the summary sheets drug companies put out and believed the relative statistics were, well, absolute.

If you went to your investment broker and he told you the return on an investment was 50 percent, whereas in absolute terms it was only 1 percent, you would no doubt sue the broker on the basis of fraud. And you would win. What we have in the cancer industry is fraud going on every day with patients who are desperate for the truth. Instead of the truth, what they get are manipulated lies.

Patients are not statisticians. The only numbers that make any sense to them are absolute numbers,[7] which stand on their own and are not *relative* to anything, but the plain, commonsensical, truth.

Unfortunately, because the effectiveness of cancer treatments is so pathetic, the industry has resorted to statistical tricks in order to turn a profit and, in my opinion, violated the doctrine of informed consent because they did not disclose the true risks involved in the treatment. In fact, they are deliberately hiding the risks behind manipulated numbers.

If you think I'm making this all up, look at the American Cancer Society's Facts and Figures booklet. It's available from their web site in .PDF format. Download the booklet and search for one instance of the word "absolute." I did this for the 2007 version and could not find a single instance. Now, search for the word "relative." You will find this word in front of every single statistic presented, but with no explanation of what "relative" means, much less what those numbers are relative to, i.e., what they are based on.

The ACS claims they are helping cancer patients, but what they are doing is helping the cancer industry[8] by deceiving patients who read their literature. The

---

[7] CA Cancer J Clin 2004;54;123-124.

same can be said for your oncologist because he or she should know better. This deception is used in all treatments, as well as diagnostic procedures, from surgery, radiation and chemotherapy to mammograms in order to justify their use.[9]

And it's not just cancer treatments. You can take *any* study of virtually *any* drug and the effectiveness of that drug will be manipulated into relative statistics by the drug company selling it. Fosamax, for example, is a drug that is supposed to reduce the risk of hip bone fractures in women. The maker claims a 44 percent reduction when taking the drug for four years. This is a big fat lie, a dishonest relative number. The absolute number? Just 1.7 percent![10] Again, a sugar pill would be more effective.

What *you* must do is ask your doctor out of 100 people, how many will benefit from the treatment? Then ask what the benefit is? How many extra days or months will a person survive with this treatment? If he or she gives you inflated numbers – if those numbers sound too good to be true, in light of what you've read thus far, then they probably are. I'd be looking for another opinion.

The bottom line: Don't trust *any* number used by the cancer industry or any company selling a drug or other medical treatment.[11]

---

[8] In 1992, the ACS aggressively recruited 16,000 healthy women into 5-year clinical trial of the chemotherapy drug Tamoxifen to the benefit of the drug maker, which financially supports the ACS. The women were told the drug was completely lsafe, despite the fact it has over 40 side effects, including cancers and both the World Health Organization and the state of California have formally designated Tamoxifen a human carcinogen! There has been no subsequent investigation with these women who were used as guinea pigs for the drug maker. The ACS was also involved with over 300,000 women in a clinical trial of high-dose mammography, despite the fact there was little evidence of the effectiveness of mammography in premenopausal women and no warnings were given to the women about the well-known high risks of breast cancer from the excessive x-ray doses that were used. The ACS has a long history of looking out for the cancer industry, not the cancer patient.

[9] This is also done with drug company advertisements, which express the benefits of a drug using deceptive relative numbers, while showing the side effects in absolute numbers, to downplay them.

[10] Resisting the Broken Bone Businesses: Bone Mineral Density Tests and the Drugs That Follow, The McDougall Newsletter, October, 2004.

[11] If cancer patients were to read the actual laboratory reports on the drugs they are taking, they would throw them away. They show neither safety nor effectiveness and, in fact, they are not intended to show either. The reports only establish a *ratio* of those who benefited from the drug and those who did not – and that ratio is usually only in the range of a few people out of a hundred. And "benefit" can mean any slight improvement, such as a temporary reduction in tumor size. If anything is proven, it is that FDA-approved cancer therapies are both unsafe and ineffective. FDA approved simply means that drug companies have complied with testing protocols – often set by the drug companies themselves and adopted by the FDA – conducted the tests and the FDA has given its

"At your next dinner party, try playing the following game. Challenge everyone around the table to produce a single drug that can cure people of an illness, other than antibiotics. If you come up with anything, stop whatever you are doing and call me."
– Lynne McTaggart

Despite the glaring failure of treatments, why would oncologists keep administering these treatments? One leading oncologist came right out and stated that the purpose of chemo is to function like a placebo in the slim hope it might work, and keep patients away from any alternative treatment:

> *"...chemotherapy serves an extremely valuable role in keeping patients oriented toward proper medical therapy.... Judicious employment and screening of potentially useful drugs may also prevent the spread of cancer quackery.... Properly based chemotherapy can serve a useful purpose in preventing improper orientation of the patient."*[12]

Dr. Jeffrey Tobias, clinical director of the Meyerstein Institute of Oncology, has said that sometimes oncologists use chemotherapy indiscriminately with "no justification other than the physician's desire to do something." Because they don't know what else to do. Other doctors have admitted using it on patients just to keep their morale up – so it looks like they are doing something. I mean, after all, if you have cancer, not only the patient, but friends and relatives all want the doctor to do something – anything! And, of course, chemo makes it appear as if the doctor is doing something. Because of that, everyone thinks the doctor is a powerful medicine man. The drug makes the patient throw up, makes them feel like they want to die and the patient's hair even falls out. The family is reassured that their doctor, for sure, is not just sitting around doing nothing! Unfortunately, they think he's in the process of curing the disease, whereas in fact he's in the process of killing the patient.

What an outrageous and cruel abuse of patients' rights. The oncologist not only gives the patient an extraordinarily toxic drug, but he lies to them about the treatment's effectiveness!

---

approval, in spite of dismal results. The real clinical trial begins when the drug is sold to the public.

[12] Victor Richards, The Wayward Cancer Cell.

"Many medical oncologists recommend chemotherapy for virtually any tumor, with a hopefulness undiscouraged by almost invariable failures."[13] – Albert Braverman, M.D., professor of oncology, State University of New York

Of course, oncologists will happily administer the drugs (except to themselves or their own family members[14]). About 75 percent of the profit for an average oncologist is made on chemotherapy drugs administered in his or her office. Given that oncologists, like other doctors, are inundated by drug company sales people, it is little wonder that chemo is given to *80 percent* of all cancer patients in the U.S., [15] despite the fact it's only somewhat effective in a very small percent of cases. In other words, we have known for decades how ineffective chemo is, yet its use has exploded.

It's become so bad that chemo is even given to patients who have been declared terminal and in their death beds! One study[16] has shown that such "treatment" either sped up or actually caused the death of 25 percent of these poor souls and 40 percent suffered significant poisoning from the treatment – not to mention sending their quality of life to hell and back during the last days of their existence.

Of course, mindlessly giving chemo to terminal patients is one reason sales of chemotherapy have continued their upward spiral until today worldwide sales are over $30 billion a year. If you don't think this is about money, open your eyes! If it were not about money, chemo would only be used on the small number of cancers where it is somewhat effective. Instead, it's used on the vast majority of cancers where it has been proven to be ineffective – and its use is justified with dishonest, distorted, rubber numbers. And while this relentless increase in chemo use continues, it's accompanied by a relentless increase in both cancer incidence and death rates, which parallel each other and reveal that the treatment strategy is simply not working – except for those who profit from such treatments.

No other branch of medicine, no other industry, has such a dismal "success" record for a standard treatment which literally affects the life and death of millions of people. How can they get away with using treatments that don't

---

[13] The Lancet, April 1991.337:901.

[14] Several surveys have been done with oncologists. A recent survey of the 64 oncologists on the staff at McGill Cancer Therapy Center in Montreal found that 91% of them said they would not take chemotherapy or allow their family members to take it for cancer treatment. Why not? It's too toxic and not effective. Yet it is apparently not too toxic or ineffective for their patients.

[15] Questioning Chemotherapy, Ralph Moss, p. 75.

[16] For Better, For Worse?, National Confidential Enquiry into Patient Outcome and Death (2008). www.ncepod.org.uk. Although this study was done on patients in Britain, the treatment practices in the U.S. are similar.

work? Because they have deliberately and systematically eliminated all other treatments that work better, but are not profitable.[17]

Results of Nutritional Therapy

"The National Cancer Institute, with enthusiastic support from the American Cancer Society...has effectively blocked funding for research and clinical trials on promising non-toxic alternative cancer drugs for decades, in favor of highly toxic and largely ineffective patented drugs developed by the multibillion dollar global cancer drug industry." – Samuel S. Epstein, M.D., The Politics of Cancer

The cancer industry has not only spent a lot of effort suppressing alternative treatments,[18] but in denying funds to study them.[19] There are a few exceptions, however. In 1995, the Office of Technological Assessment (OTA) did a retrospective study of five-year survival rates for melanoma patients who were given nutritional treatments versus conventional therapy. The results were very impressive compared to conventional therapy.[20]

---

[17] See the film "Healing Cancer From Inside Out" by Mike Anderson.

[18] Two books which document some of the effective natural cures for cancer which have come along in the past 75 years – and have faced a tidal wave of opposition from the cancer industry – are The Cancer Industry by Ralph Moss and Options by Richard Walters.

[19] The NCI's medical standards should be called a double standard when applied to alternative treatments. For example, when a *single* patient in a clinical setting responds to a new chemotherapy drug, this is sometimes considered sufficient cause to launch clinical trials, as happened in the study of Interleukin. Alternative practitioners, on the other hand, have been required to supply massive documentation of benefit and safety before even the most preliminary tests can be approved. The standard for safety is equally elastic, especially considering the extreme toxicity of chemo drugs and radiation, in contrast with the relative harmlessness of almost all the alternative therapies. I personally know of one doctor whose alternative treatment is undergoing clinical trials to get FDA approval. Despite the object harassment by the FDA, the treatment has passed all trials with flying colors, to date. Under pressure from pharmaceutical companies, the FDA is now requiring him to add chemotherapy to his protocol. The treatment is completely non-toxic and adding chemo will ruin it – exactly what the drug companies are trying to accomplish.

[20] Gar Hildenbrand et al., "Five-Year Survival Rates of Melanoma Patients Treated by Diet Therapy After the Manner of Gerson: A Retrospective Review," Alternative Therapies, Sept 1995, p. 29.

Percent 5-Year Survival

	Nutritional Therapy	Conventional Therapy
Melanoma Stage IIIA	82%	39%
Melanoma Stage IVA	39%	6%

A 15-year retrospective survey on the outcome of nutritional treatments with patients suffering from malignant melanoma revealed the following five-year survival rates:[21]

	Percent 5-Year Survival
Stages I & II (localized)	100%
Stage III (regional spread)	71%
Stage IVA (superficial distant spread)	39%

Although not compared directly with conventional treatments, these results far exceed – by a huge margin – what can be expected from any conventional treatment of melanoma.

A study[22] was done with pancreatic cancer patients who were divided into two groups. The first group made no dietary changes and 99 percent were dead within a year. The second group consumed a moderately healthy plant-based diet and 52 percent were alive after a year.

Over the course of six years, the more vegetables lung cancer patients ate, the longer they lived.[23] The more vegetables colon cancer patients ate, the longer they lived.[24]

In a study by the National Cancer Institute[25], women were divided into two groups. The first group stayed on their typical American diets and the second group changed to a plant-based diet. After only four years, almost 40 percent of the women on typical diets had recurrences of breast cancer. *Not a single woman* who changed to a plant-based diet had a recurrence of breast cancer.

Women who simply ate flaxseed muffins on a daily basis had a reduction in breast tumors equivalent to those taking the toxic drug Tamoxifen – and without any side effects.[26] (This is not to say that simply eating flaxseed muffins are all

---

[21] For detailed documentation, visit www.gerson-research.org/docs/HildenbrandGLG-1995-1/index.html.

[22] J Amer Coll Nutr, 12:3:209-215; Macrobiotic Diet and Cancer Survival, JP Carter, J Amer Coll Nutr, 12:3:209-215, 1993.

[23] Eur J CA, 28: 2: 45; Goodman, MT, Vegetable consumption in lung cancer longevity, Eur J CA, 28: 2: 45-499, 1992.

[24] JAMA. 2007 Aug 15; 298(7):754-64.

[25] Journal of the National Cancer Institute, January, 1993.

[26] Biological Effects of Dietary Flaxseed In Patients With Breast Cancer, Thompson LU, Li T, Chen J, Goss PE Nutritional Sciences, University of Toronto, Toronto, ON,

that effective against breast tumors because Tamoxifen is not at all effective, either! It is to say, why take Tamoxifen when muffins are just as good?)

Women who switched to low-fat diets had their estrogen levels drop by up to 50 percent within a few weeks.[27] Women with early stage breast cancer who changed to a slightly healthy plant-based diet – combined with exercise – cut their risk of death in half.[28]

Researchers compared health and diet histories among two groups — 541 women who had endometrial cancer, and a matched number of women who had no history of cancer. The results showed that women with the highest amount of vegetables in their diets had a 50 percent lower risk of endometrial cancer than those with the lowest vegetable intake.[29]

A recent study of stage III colon cancer patients showed that those people who adopted a slightly healthier diet with higher intakes of plant foods, lived three times longer than those who did not.[30]

A change to a full plant-based diet inhibited the growth of prostate cancer cells by almost eight times, compared to the control group.[31]

A study found that the median survival time for men with prostate cancer, who received aggressive treatment, was just six years. The median survival time

---

Canada; Medical Oncology, Princess Margaret Hospital, Toronto, ON, Canada, San Antonio Breast Cancer Symposium 2000. Regarding side effects, Tamoxifen increases the risk of endometrial cancer, blood clots in the legs, dangerous blockage of arteries in the lungs (pulmonary embolism), and stroke, to name just a few.

[27] JAMA, 2005; vol. 293: p 2479; Prentice R, et al. Dietary fat reduction and plasma estradiol concentration in healthy postmenopausal women. The Women's Health Trial Study Group. J Natl Cancer Inst. 1990;82:129-134; Heber D, et al. Reduction of serum estradiol in postmenopausal women given free access to low-fat high-carbohydrate diet. Nutrition. 1991;7:137-139.

[28] Pierce, J.P. Journal of Clinical Oncology, Jun 10, 2007; online edition. John P. Pierce, PhD, Cancer Prevention and Control Program, Moores USCD Cancer Center, University of California, San Diego. The Journal of the American Medical Association, 2005; vol 293: pp 2479-2486. American Cancer Society: "Low-Fat Diet May Stall Breast Cancer Recurrence."

[29] Yeh M, et al. Higher intakes of vegetables and vegetable-related nutrients are associated with lower endometrial cancer risks. The Journal of Nutrition. December 11, 2008 [Epub date]

[30] Meyerhardt JA, Niedzwiecki D, Hollis D, Saltz LB, Hu FB, Mayer RJ, Nelson H, Whittom R, Hantel A, Thomas J, Fuchs CS. Association of dietary patterns with cancer recurrence and survival in patients with stage III colon cancer. JAMA. 2007 Aug 15;298(7):754-64.

[31] J Urol 2005;174:1065-1070. See also Frattaroli J, Weidner G, Dnistrian AM, Kemp C, Daubenmier JJ, Marlin RO, Crutchfield L, Yglecias L, Carroll PR, Ornish D. Clinical events in prostate cancer lifestyle trial: results from two years of follow-up. Urology. 2008 Dec;72(6):1319-23.

for men with prostate cancer who did not receive any treatment – and changed to a plant-based diet – was 19 years![32]

The Kushi Institute presented to the National Institutes of Health detailed documentation on six cases of terminally ill cancer patients who reversed their cancers by adopting a plant-based diet.[33] This is what Ralph Moss, a well-known reporter in the cancer field, said of their documentation:

> *"A nurse told how, in 1995, she was diagnosed with lung cancer that had spread all over her body. She received no effective conventional therapy, and reluctantly went on the macrobiotics diet...What makes this case so extraordinary is that her progress was monitored weekly by a sympathetic physician colleague. The shrinkage, and finally the disappearance, of her tumors was documented millimeter by millimeter! She has now been disease-free for over five years..."[34]*

In fact, all of the people who reversed their cancers have survived far longer than five years and at the time of this writing are alive and well, despite the fact conventional medicine said they should be dead.

The Cancer Advisory Panel on Complimentary and Alternative Medicine (CAPCAM), which studied these cases, recommended funding for additional study of nutritional treatments. Guess what? It never came. Guess what? It never will, so long as conventional medicine has a stranglehold on our medical mindset. This has been the problem from the beginning. Back in 1946, Dr. Max Gerson presented six of his own terminal cases (which he reversed with diet) before a Senate subcommittee and funding was denied based on heavy lobbying from medical interests, particularly the AMA.[35]

When your doctor says there's no "scientific" evidence of diet reversing cancers, what he or she means is that there has been no large-scale, peer-reviewed study published in the New England Journal of Medicine. Of course there hasn't! There have been many attempts to get funding for such studies, but such attempts have always been vigorously opposed by medical interests. (By the

---

[32] James Carter et al., "Hypothesis: Dietary Management May Improve Survival From Nutritionally Linked Cancers..." Journal of the American College of Nutrition, 12(2), 1993, PP. 209-26; James Carter et al., "Cancers With Suspected Nutritional Links: Dietary Management?" Tulane University School of Public Health and Tropical Medicine, Feb 1990; See also: Journal of the American College of Nutrition, 12(3), 1993, pp. 209-26.

[33] The cancers were lung, non-Hodgkin's lymphoma, ovarian, malignant melanoma, pancreas-lymph nodes-liver and breast. www.kushiinstitute.org/html/government.html.

[34] Moss Reports Newsletter, Feb 27, 2002.

[35] For a short history of the Gerson Therapy written by the US Office of Technology Assessment, see http://gerson-research.org/docs/WardPS-1988-1/index.html#GersonM-1945-1.

way, if you have some extra cash and wish to fund such a study, please contact me.)

Philip E. Binzel, Jr., M.D., has meticulously documented the outcomes of treating his own cancer patients with diet and natural supplementation. He compared his results to those shown by the American Cancer Society for conventional treatments.[36] (Primary cancer is defined as detectable cancer confined to a single area, with perhaps a few adjacent lymph nodes involved. Metastatic cancer is defined as a cancer located in multiple areas of the body.)

Patient Survival (5 years or more)

	Nutritional Therapy	Conventional Therapy
Primary Cancer	87%*	15%
Metastatic Cancer	70%	0.1%

* Did not die of cancer and survived more than 18 years.

Although the studies on treating cancer with nutrition are infrequent, the data is overwhelmingly positive, showing that diet can have a profound and lasting effect. They also show that when it comes to curing cancer, nutritional treatments are far more effective than conventional treatments.[37] And there are literally thousands of documented cases of people reversing all stages of all types of cancers. Why hasn't this been more thoroughly studied?

The effectiveness of nutritional treatments scares conventional medicine and explains why they have fought so hard to deny funding for further study of diet. They are so anxious to protect their profitable, toxic and ineffective treatments they have even rigged studies on dietary treatments and natural supplementation

---

[36] Alive and Well, Philip E. Binzel, Jr., M.D., p. 107.

[37] There may be some readers thinking this is all bunk because the gold standard for testing is double-blind, randomized, placebo-controlled testing. Well, first of all, that rarely happens with any cancer drug these days. Here's what Ralph Moss has said about it: "In fact, true placebo controls have been almost abandoned in the testing of chemotherapy. Drug regimen is tested against drug regimen, and doctors hardly every look at whether the drugs do better than simple good nursing care. The value of chemotherapy is a given." (Ralph Moss, Questioning Chemotherapy, p. 57) Secondly, such tests may be appropriate for simple-minded, tumor-targeted testing, but they are highly inappropriate for dietary treatments which affect the entire body, not just a localized part of the body (e.g., looking for tumor response rates). Response rates of a tumor are irrelevant to dietary treatments and tumor shrinkage may well lag behind the rest of the body as it heals itself. In other words, the focus of dietary treatments is the whole body, not just a tumor. An appropriate test would be to take two groups with the same cancer, at the same stage. One group follows conventional treatments and the other a *true* anti-cancer diet. My money says the latter group will have many more survivors. In every test like this, dietary treatments win.

so they were doomed to fail.[38] Why are they so afraid? They are scared that people will abandon conventional treatments and flock to clinics which use dietary treatments. And they're right. If you had a choice between following a strict diet or chemotherapy, I can pretty much guess which choice you would make. If everyone knew just how ineffective conventional treatments really are, the choice would be a no-brainer.

The point is that the cancer industry has to manipulate statistics and clinical trials[39] in order to make their treatments look better than what you would expect by taking a sugar pill.

---

[38] See *Part 3 – Laetrile.*

[39] Clinical trials are supposed to be the "gold standard" of scientific study, and yet it has been well demonstrated that these studies almost always produce results beneficial to the organization providing the funding, which is anxious to turn a buck. The wishes of the study sponsors, not true scientific methods, almost always determine study outcomes. This is accomplished through an elaborate system of fraudulent trial design, selective reporting, dismissing study subjects who don't produce the desired outcomes, statistical distortions and the application of career pressure to the researchers who carry out such studies. (Researchers who don't produce the desired results get fired or blackballed by the industry.) As Marsha Angell, former editor of the New England Journal of Medicine, has said, "[Clinical] trials can be rigged in a dozen ways and it happens all the time." During clinical trials, it's not all that uncommon for patients to die, yet they are not reported as dead. In fact, dead people have been listed as subjects for testing. Often, people are not in the hospital during the times of the tests and yet they are recorded as having been in the test. It's been discovered that patient consent forms bore dates showing the subjects were dead before they supposedly signed the form. Another trick is to replace patients who died, with other patients replacements, without changing the records in order to conceal the deaths. I'm not saying this is the norm, but it does point out that drug companies will do anything they can to put the best face on a drug. A more common practice, in clinical trials, is to count a control patient who dies of any cause as a failure of non-treatment, whereas a patient who dies just before a treatment program is completed, is not counted as a failure of treatment on the grounds that the patient had not completed the treatment program! One study by the FDA itself showed that one in five doctors researching the effects of new drugs had simply invented the data they reported and pocketed the fees. Or a study may start with 100 people and end up with 70 – yet no explanation is given (or required) to explain what happened to the 30 people who were dropped from the rolls. Perhaps the more egregious and common practice is that reports showing unfavorable results are rarely published and clinicians, of course, are pressured into keeping quiet about these unpublished studies. These are just some of the reasons why we learn about the true nature of a drug after it's been on the market for years – and killed many people. There are thousands of drugs that have been approved by the FDA because they were supposedly proven to cure or prevent a disease – as well as being safe and effective. Then years later, they were taken off the market because 1) they were shown not to cure or prevent a disease or 2) they had such terrible side effects they were too dangerous for people to use. In fact, the true test subjects for drug companies are the public.

A Tumor Fetish

"Although cancer appears to strike suddenly, often without warning, it does not happen overnight. Rather, it is a slow, steady progression that [often] takes literally up to 40 years to reveal itself." – Robert Hatherill, Ph.D.

"Surgery is really not a 'cure'. Rather it's an amputation of the problem. It doesn't say anything about solving it, but simply eliminates the symptom."
– Ralph Moss, Ph.D., author of The Cancer Industry

"...tumor regression by itself is actually a lousy predictor....regression is not likely to improve a person's chances of survival."
– Dr. Robert Weinberg, Massachusetts Institute of Technology

The awareness of cancer begins, in most cases, with the discovery of a tumor, either by the individual or by screening. The tumor, however, is only a symptom of a disease which, in almost all cases, has been growing in the body for many, many years – it's just the tip of the iceberg.

So what do you do? You go to an oncologist. Oncology is, after all, the study of tumors. And by definition, seeing an oncologist is seeing someone about a symptom of cancer, someone who can treat a symptom, but not the disease itself. Their focus is the tumor so it's little surprise that when oncologists see a patient, he will ask, "How's the tumor doing?" without ever asking how the patient is doing.

If you want to stump your oncologist, ask him, "What caused the cancer?" The answer will invariably be "We don't know."

This state of knowledge greatly limits treatment options and explains why treating a symptom has become an obsession. When presented with such limited treatment options, the patient will often say "Oh, just get rid of the damn thing!" And the oncologist will happily begin slashing, burning and poisoning in an effort to get rid of the tumor, without ever attempting to treat the underlying cause of it.

With only a few rare exceptions, tumors are neither health-endangering nor life-threatening. In some cases, surgical removal of a tumor can be beneficial, if it has grown to such a size that it is blocking or interfering with bodily functions. But again, this is a temporary fix and does not solve the underlying problem.

Taking off breasts in radical mastectomy reminds me of when doctors took out tonsils, because they did not understand what they were doing. By surgically removing actress Christina Applegate's breasts, for example, cancer surgeons have misled her into thinking she's cured, when in reality, she still has the exact same risk of cancer as she did before the surgery. This is because if a woman truly has breast cancer, the disease has already spread to the rest of her body, under the radar, long before the breast cancer was diagnosed.[40] No matter how much of her anatomy she removes, the underlying cause of the cancer is still with her.

As Dr. Todd Tuttle has stated,[41]

"I'm afraid that women believe having their opposite breast removed is somehow going to improve their breast cancer survival. In fact, it probably will not affect their survival."

Destroying a beehive, in other words, does not get rid of the bees – and they'll create another hive in time, somewhere else, to replace the one that has been destroyed. The real tragedy is that doctors have convinced Christina she is out of the woods and there is nothing more to do. In her words, "I'm clear. Absolutely 100 percent clear and clean. It did not spread – they got everything out, so I'm definitely not going to die from breast cancer."[42] This may sound familiar to those of you who remember when the doctors declared Farrah Fawcett (and so many others) "clear" of cancer, only to have it return.

In most cases, the focus is on tumor *shrinkage*, not removal. In fact, the FDA approves chemotherapy drugs if the drug can shrink a tumor by 50 percent or more within 28 days. The problem is that there is no relationship between tumor shrinkage and extending the life of the patient. Why should there be? They are only attacking a symptom of a disease that is still active in the body. Tumor shrinkage – or removal – has absolutely no effect on the underlying conditions that allowed this abnormal growth to thrive in the first place.

A famous case of wonderful tumor shrinkage was former Senator Hubert Humphrey, who was treated with radiation for his bladder cancer. The treatment was so effective that three years after it began his physician, Willard Whitmore, M.D., declared, "As far as we are concerned, the Senator is cured." Despite the cure declaration, they began treating the senator with chemotherapy. Shortly after treatment began, Senator Humphrey called chemo "bottled death." His words were not only correct, but also prophetic. He was dead within a year, despite the fact he had been "cured."

Of course, you're probably saying, "That was a long time ago. Treatments have improved since then." I'm here to tell you they have not. And life-expectancy rates (long-term survival) following treatments have not budged one iota. The reason? Chemo and radiation both work by killing rapidly dividing cells. Unfortunately, rapidly dividing cancer cells only occur in a very small

---

[40] Journal of Surg Onc 1997 Aug 65 (4) 284-97.
[41] Tuttle TM, et al. Use of Contralateral Prophylactic Mastectomy for Breast Cancer Patients: A Trend Toward More Aggressive Surgical Treatment. J Clin Oncol. 2007 October 22.
[42] Applegate Underwent Breast Removal to Stop Cancer, ABC News, Aug. 19, 2008 www.abcnews.go.com/GMA/story?id=5606034.

number of cancers (the very same reason chemo is somewhat effective in only a small number of cancers). In all other cases, cancer cells actually have slower division rates than the most active cells of the body. Thus, it is biologically impossible for chemo to work without doing significant damage to other parts of body. As a result, the strategy adopted by conventional medicine is to try to kill the cancer, before the treatment kills the patient. In the case of Senator Humphrey – and millions of others – that strategy did (and does) not work.

A more recent example is Tony Snow, the former White House Press Secretary, who was diagnosed initially with colon cancer and, after treatment, died when the cancer was detected in his liver and other areas of his body. The surgery they performed on him severely restricted his normal eliminative functions, which overburdened his liver and tissue fluids with toxic waste. The previous series of chemo treatments impaired his immune system and weakened him greatly. Did the cancer do this to him? Of course not – the treatments did! Between the chemo and surgery, these two treatments created a perfect recipe for creating new cancers – and that is exactly what happened. Once again, more harm than good was done by the treatments.

You don't have to go to an oncologist to get tumor shrinkage. You can do it yourself at home. Just start injecting rat poison into your veins. It will make you vomit, attack every organ in your body, make you feel like you want to die, and your hair will no doubt fall out. It produces all the wonderful side effects of chemo, and it's a lot less expensive. Think I'm kidding? Rat poison was recently found in tainted pet food, which was killing cats and dogs. The substance in the rat poison that killed them? Aminopterin, a cancer drug.[43]

Your doctor may bring up the subject of a treatment having great response rates (shrinkage) for tumors, but the doctor is setting up unrealistic hopes for the patient because response rates have nothing to do with how long you will live. So your tumor shrank due to radiation and chemo.[44] Big deal. What your doctors probably won't tell you is that your heart, liver and kidneys were damaged at the same time. The tumor shrinks, but you get sicker and sicker because of the treatment. Now, you're going to need prescription drugs, probably for the rest of your life. The treatment makes you so sick that you need other treatments to offset the effects of the first treatment; and perhaps a second round of drugs to offset the effects of the drugs prescribed to you for the initial treatment – and on down the line. All of a sudden, your body has become a chemistry lab and physicians are trying to balance all the side effects of all the drugs you are on, while those drugs are busy destroying your body.

---

[43] AP, 3/24/07, www.msnbc.msn.com/id/17754681/ Of course, the government currently prohibits using aminopterin in rat poison, but it's Ok to inject it in humans – and it's still used in other countries to kill rodents.

[44] Over time, cancer cells often develop drug-resistance and the drugs are unable to shrink the tumor.

The obsession with tumor shrinkage is rather strange. Tumor shrinkage is really not a big deal. When you attack the underlying cause of the cancer, tumors will shrink – and without surgery, chemotherapy or radiation. That is, conventional treatments do not have a monopoly on tumor shrinkage. Just as your arm may swell temporarily due to an injury, the swelling subsides as your body heals. And so it is with tumors. As you heal your entire body, it reverses the conditions that allow tumors to thrive. (See *Part 2 – Reversing Cancer.*)

I recently received a letter from a woman with breast cancer, who opted to follow my dietary strategy instead of conventional treatment. After a couple of weeks on the diet, she exclaimed, almost in disbelief, "My tumor is shrinking!!" Please don't "disbelieve" this can happen. When you attack the underlying cause of any disease, the symptoms of the disease go away. In the case of cancer, that symptom most often happens to be a tumor.

It should be noted that on nutritional therapy, the tumor won't necessarily disappear in all cases. Once a tumor has become firmly established in the body, the body will accept it as normal tissue and not attack it. A tumor is comprised of many different components and usually is no more than 10 percent cancerous, anyway.[45] When this happens, the tumor can be removed for cosmetic reasons.

There is nothing in surgery, radiation or chemotherapy that will prevent the spread of cancer. In the end, it is not localized tumors that kill people, it's the spread of cancer cells to the bones, liver, lungs, brain or other vital areas – until the cancer overtakes the body. The idea that you can somehow "contain" cancer cells in one part of the body – without being able to detect *all* cancer cells in the body (those "under the radar") – is moronic. It's not the tumor, but the conditions inside the body that promote cancer and allow it to thrive and spread.

It's a very odd mindset which thinks that by attacking a symptom, you can cure a disease. This is why recurrence rates are so high. It's laughable, really, because long-term cures are almost by accident – not the result of the treatment – and usually the result of the patient taking charge of their health and doing something on their own. They are cured despite the treatment, not because of it. (In fact, according to one expert only about one percent of patients in clinical trials ever develops complete remission![46])

Now, let's imagine that through conventional methods, a tumor shrinks significantly over a period of six months, but the patient dies in the seventh month. The cancer industry would classify the treatment as a success – because the yardstick for success is, after all, tumor shrinkage.

Conversely, suppose a patient with a similar tumor is treated with nutrition. And suppose he is alive after two years, but the tumor is no smaller. The cancer industry would classify that treatment as a failure – because the tumor did not get any smaller!

---

[45] Alive and Well, Philip E. Binzel, Jr., M.D., p. 136.
[46] Questioning Chemotherapy, Ralph Moss, pp. 64-65.

In other words, the cancer industry is primarily interested in whether the tumor gets bigger or smaller – because the condition of a symptom is their yardstick for success. To destroy trillions of healthy cells and your immune system with toxic treatments just to get a billion-cell tumor is like using dynamite to kill a mouse in your kitchen.

Gout is a disease that attacks the joints. But we do not amputate a hand or leg to treat it. We treat the underlying cause of the disease (most effectively with diet). The swelling and pain in the joints is simply a symptom of the disease.

The real tragedy is that after a tumor is removed and the patient "cured," another tumor will most likely appear in another part of the body after a few years because the treatment has done nothing to bolster the body's own defense systems and everything to destroy them. Within a year, the cancer regains its powers and starts growing, long before the debilitated immune system is strong enough to combat the illness. This is why up to 70 percent of women with breast cancer – who had the cancer show up in their lymph nodes – die from the illness. Their immune systems were wiped out as a result of the treatment and could not contain the spreading cancer.

Screening for Dollars

"Marketing a disease is the best way to market a drug." – Susan Love, M.D.

"...Mammograms increase the risk for developing breast cancer and raise the risk of spreading or metastasizing an existing growth." – Charles B. Simone, M.D., former clinical associate in immunology and pharmacology at the National Cancer Institute

"...the annual mammographic screening of 10,000 women aged 50-70 will extend the lives of, at best, 26 of them; and annual screening of 10,000 women in their 40s will extend the lives of only 12 women per year."
– "How Mammography Causes Cancer," Alternative Medicine, Sep. 1999

"Of every 1,000 American women getting mammograms each year between the ages of 40 and 50, 345 [35%] will receive false positive results, often with unnecessary intervention [i.e., treatment] as the result." – New England Journal of Medicine, February 11, 1993

"...a truthful account of the facts must be available to the public and the individual patient. It will not be what they want to hear." – M. Maureen Roberts, Clinical Director, Edinburgh Breast Cancer Screening Project

Early detection has been the clarion call of the cancer industry, which gets massive numbers of people into the system in hopes of finding that almighty tumor. In effect, early detection is "early recruitment" of patients into treatment procedures which any other business would have abandoned years ago because they are so ineffective – except for the fact that these treatments still bring billions of dollars into the industry.

Sometimes, early detection will catch a fast-growing tumor, but this is so rare your chances of being struck by lightning are better. In almost all cases, screening detects slow growing tumors that do not have to be acted on right away. By the time a tumor is large enough to be detected by mammography, it's been there for at least a decade. In other words, advertising mammography as "early detection" is ludicrous and simply a PR stunt by the industry.

One of the main arguments used to justify regular screening is that women who get regular screenings live longer. What's never mentioned is exactly how much how longer they live.

Many studies say the same thing when looking at this longevity benefit. Let's take one from The Lancet[47] which shows that this much-ballyhooed life extension boils down not to years or months, but just a few days of extra life.

The Benefits of Regular Mammograms

Woman in her 40s:	3 extra days in her life
Woman in her 50s:	4 extra days in her life
Woman in her 60s:	9 extra days in her life

These, of course, are absolute numbers and you will find similar numbers in virtually every study that has ever been done – once you translate the rubber numbers into honest ones.

If you put cancer industry spin on these numbers, however, the relative numbers translate into a whopping 20 percent longevity benefit. When the public hears there's a 20 percent benefit to getting regular mammograms, the average

---

[47] The Lancet, 355, Jan 8, 2000; 355:80-81; an updated review of the study can be found in The Lancet,359, Mar 16, 2002; 904-905. The relative death benefit of 20 percent is based on the determination that out of 129,750 women who were invited to begin having mammograms in the late 1970s and early 1980s, 511 died of breast cancer over the next 15 years – a death rate of 0.4 percent. In the comparison group of 117,260 women, who were not invited, there were 584 breast cancer deaths over the same period – a death rate of 0.5 percent. The difference between 0.4 percent and 0.5 percent translates into a 20 percent *relative* benefit in favor of mammography. But the absolute difference between the two groups after eight years of mammography is only seven deaths a year in a female population of 250,000! In other words, the absolute difference is ZERO. And that seemingly wonderful 20 percent relative benefit translates into only a few additional days of life for all age groups. For a good discussion of just how absurd relative numbers are, see Should I Be Tested for Cancer, H. Gilbert Welch, M.D., M.P.H., pp. 23-26.

women is going to think, "Gosh, that's going to extend my life by 20 percent!" She then grabs her coat and heads down to the hospital for her annual dose of radiation.

But as Donald Barry, the chief of biostatistics at the M.D. Anderson Cancer Center has said:[48]

> "[Relative benefit] is OK for statistical inferences, but it is meaningless for a woman making a screen decision. **_Absolute risk reduction is what matters_**." (emphasis added)

Let's illustrate this industry spin with a simple example. Suppose that *four* women out of one million – who did not get mammograms – developed breast cancer, but only *three* women – who did get mammograms – developed breast cancer. In absolute terms, the difference is only one person *out of a million* (i.e., zero). That's not only statistically insignificant, it's statistically absurd. The relative benefit, however, would be a whopping 25 percent reduction in the chances of developing breast cancer (three women vs. four women). And this is exactly what the cancer industry advertises to naïve women: a big fat lie.

When doctors explain benefits in absolute (honest) terms, few women choose to get mammograms. In fact, two noted researchers recommended the withdrawal of public funding for mammograms altogether.

> "The benefit is marginal, the harm caused is substantial, and the costs incurred are enormous, [so] we suggest that public funding for breast cancer screening in any age group is not justifiable."
> – Drs. Wright and Mueller[49]

One study, in fact, showed a 52 percent *increase* in breast cancer in women under 50 who were given annual mammograms.[50] In women under 40, the increase in breast cancer has gone up 3,000 percent since widespread mammography began. It's also been estimated that the painful compression of breast tissue during mammograms can increase the possibility of metastasis by as much as 80 percent![51]

Since mammography was introduced in 1983, the incidence of ductal carcinoma in-situ (DCIS), which now represents 12 percent of all breast cancer cases, has increased by 328 percent for women of all ages and 200 percent of this increase is due to mammograms.[52] For women under 40, DCIS has gone up over

---

[48] Statistics misleading, some doctors say relative numbers skew benefit to look much larger, Chicago Tribune, March 15, 2002.
[49] The Lancet, July 1, 1995.
[50] The Politics of Cancer Revisited, Samuel S. Epstein, M.D., p. 351.
[51] The McDougall Program for Women, John A. McDougall, M.D., p 105.
[52] The Lancet, July 1, 1995; Under The Influence Modern Medicine by Terry A Rondberg DC, page 123. In addition to harmful radiation, this encapsulated, self-limiting

3,000 percent![53] Radiation-induced breast cancers normally occur at least 10 years after exposure. Radiation from yearly mammograms during the ages of 40 to 49 has been estimated to cause one additional breast cancer death per 10,000 women.[54]

The routine practice of taking four films of each breast annually results in approximately 1 rad (radiation absorbed dose) exposure, which is 1,000 times greater than what you would get from a chest X-ray. As a result, it is now estimated that annual mammograms increase the risk of breast cancer by one to two percent a year. So over a 10-year period, the cumulative risk of getting cancer from early screenings will have been increased by 10 to 20 percent!

Even worse, a recent study exposed the dangers of full-body CT scans (computerized tomography), stating that the radiation received is equal to that of 100 mammograms and similar to the radiation exposure received by survivors of the atomic bombings of Hiroshima and Nagasaki, who were about 1 1/2 miles from the explosions.[55] The authors state that radiation from one scan is enough to produce a tumor in every 1,200 people who undergo the procedure. For those who have annual scans, the risk goes as high as one tumor in every 50 people.

Even the National Cancer Institute – as well as other experts – agrees that mammograms are likely to cause more cancers than could possibly be detected. Among women under 35, mammography could cause 75 cases of breast cancer for every 15 it identifies.[56] A Canadian study found a 52 percent increase in breast cancer mortality in young women given annual mammograms.[57] And

---

and harmless cancer can spread due to the compressive force of routine mammograms. An acquaintance diagnosed with DCIS and was talked into a radical mastectomy. After they removed her breasts, they had them biopsied and – low and behold – they found cancer in other areas of her breast, aside from the encapsulated DCIS site. The doctors told her it was a good thing they removed her breasts, thus justifying the surgery. Well, of course they found cancer. They had been blasting her with radiation for years! One of the reasons she went for a radical mastectomy is because she was told that reconstructive surgery would restore her appearance and no one would ever know the difference. After a year of very painful procedures, it was finally determined she was not suitable for reconstructive surgery. She now has two missing breasts and will psychologically suffer the rest of her life as a result of surgeons aggressively going after a cancer that hardly anyone ever dies from. Due to early detection, she was aggressively treated for a "disease" that in all likelihood would never have troubled her, much less killed her. For a discussion of the debate on treating DCIS, see A Debate on How to Treat Precancerous Breast Disease, NY Times, June 22, 2004. See also, Ernster VL, Barclay J. Increase in ductal carcinoma in situ (DCIS) of the breast in relation to mammography: a dilemma. Natl Cancer Inst Monogr 1997; 22: 151-156.

[53] The Lancet, July 1, 1995.
[54] Under The Influence Modern Medicine by Terry A Rondberg DC, page 122.
[55] David J. Brenner, Carl D. Elliston. Estimated Radiation Risks Potentially Associated with Full-Body CT Screening. Radiology 2004;232:735-738.
[56] The Politics Of Cancer Revisited, Samuel S. Epstein, M.D., p. 290.
[57] Samuel S. Epstein, M.D., Cancer-Gate, p. 35.

having mammograms during pregnancy could endanger the fetus with future risks of leukemia, not to mention birth defects. Similarly, studies reveal that children exposed to radiation are more likely to develop breast cancer as adults – and the younger the woman at the time of exposure, the greater her lifetime risk for breast cancer. Worse still, researchers estimate that 10,000 women, who have a gene (oncogene AC), which makes them extremely sensitive to even small doses of radiation, will die of breast cancer this year – all as a result of the cancer industry dialing for mammogram dollars.

Here is what The Lancet said about screening in the year 2000:

> *"Screening for breast cancer with mammography is unjustified... for every 1,000 women screened...one breast-cancer death is avoided whereas the total number of deaths is increased by six.... There is no reliable evidence that screening decreases breast-cancer mortality."*[58]

Again, more harm than good and nothing has changed since then to alter that opinion.

Despite long-standing claims, the evidence that routine mammography reduces mortality is one of the biggest medical frauds being run today. In fact, the key variables predicting survival have nothing to do with early detection at all. It is the virulence of the cancer and the strength of one's immune system that count.[59]

With regard to mammograms causing cancer, it is instructive to look into what happened to Irwin D. Bross, Ph.D., former Director of Bio-Statistics at Roswell Park Memorial Institute for Cancer Research.

He discovered there are three types of cancer: benign, malignant and cancers that look malignant but are not malignant and only become malignant when exposed to radiation and drugs (i.e., chemo). He discovered that *more than half* of those diagnosed with breast cancer had *benign* lesions that were *unable to spread*! He wrote,[60]

> *"What most women have is a tumour which, under a light microscope, looks like a cancer to a pathologist. Chances are, this tumour lacks the ability to metastasise – to spread throughout the body – which is the hallmark of a genuine cancer."*

---

[58] The Lancet 2000; 355:129-134; see also BMJ. 1988 October 15; 297(6654): 943–948.
[59] Lerner, B. H. Public health then and now: Great expectations: Historical perspectives on genetic breast cancer testing, pp. 11- 13; Am. J. Public Health 89(6): 938- 944, 1999.
[60] Bross, Irwin D, 'Breast cancer: the one scientific fact you need to know'; See also NEJM 1994; 331: 809.

In other words, half the women diagnosed with breast cancer have a benign breast cancer and should not be treated at all. But when subjected to radiation and chemotherapy, that benign lesion can turn malignant, i.e., it can become a doctor-induced (iatrogenic) cancer.

Bross went on to say,

> *"Our discovery was highly unpopular with the medical profession. Doctors could never afford to admit the scientific truth because the standard treatment in those days was radical mastectomy. Admitting the truth could lead to malpractice suits by women who had lost a breast because of an incorrect medical diagnosis."*

When Dr. Bross released his findings, which linked ionizing radiation with the triggering of malignant cancer, how was he rewarded for this potentially life-saving discovery? The National Cancer Institute abruptly and unceremoniously stopped funding his work!

Bross went on to say that mammography would cause four or five cancers for every one detected, leading to[61]

> *"...the worst epidemic of iatrogenic [doctor-induced] breast cancer in history. In my view...the NCI would be better off putting the money allocated for future screenings into a trust fund for the victims of [mammograms] who will develop cancer in 10 to 15 years time."*

Recently, a study showed that women in the same age brackets who were screened every two years had higher rates of breast cancer than those who were screened every six years.[62] This not only suggests that the more frequent mammograms were causing higher rates of cancer, but that the lower cancer rates were the result of the body healing cancer on its own, given the six-year interval between screenings.[63]

---

[61] Bross, Irwin D, 'Breast cancer: the one scientific fact you need to know.

[62] Robert M. Kaplan, PhD; Franz Porzsolt, MD, PhD, The Natural History of Breast Cancer, Arch Intern Med. 2008;168(21):2302-2303.

[63] See Everson, Tilden C and Cole, Warren Henry, Spontaneous regression of cancer; a study and abstract of reports in the world medical literature and of personal communications concerning spontaneous regression of malignant disease; Kolata G, Study suggests some cancers may go away. New York Times Nov 25 2008; Miller AB, To T, Baines CJ, et al., The Canadian National Breast Screening Study-1: breast cancer mortality after 11 to 16 years of follow-up. A randomized screening trial of mammography in women age 40 to 49 years. Ann Intern Med 2002;137(5 Part 1):305-12; Mulcahy N. Mammography study suggests some breast cancer may spontaneously regress. Medscape Medical News Nov 25 2008; Zahl P-H, Strand BH, Maehlen J,

As Robert Kaplan said:[64]

> *"Perhaps the most important concern raised by the study is that it highlights how surprisingly little we know about what happens to untreated patients with breast cancer."* (See *The Do Nothing Strategy.*)

Although it is done on a daily basis, reading a mammogram is an extremely tricky business. The man who first developed the mammogram said on national television that only about six – repeat six – radiologists in the entire United States could read them correctly![65]

Your doctor, of course, will tell you that mammography is 90 percent (or more) accurate. That is simply wrong.[66] What he is using is (once again) *relative statistics*. The absolute statistic is *only nine percent*.

Approximately eight out of 1,000 women have breast cancer today. Of these eight women, seven will have a positive mammogram (true positive). Of the remaining 992 women who do not have breast cancer, 70 will have a false positive. The accuracy of the test, in other words, is $7 / (7 + 70) = 9$ percent.

If you take a second mammogram and that is positive, the accuracy would jump to around 57 percent, but that's not much better than flipping a coin. Only when you take a third test that is positive you can be reasonably certain (93%) that you have breast cancer. (And after that many tests, you'll probably glow in the dark, to boot!)

In other words, out of the total of 77 (true and false) positives discovered by mammography, only seven will be correct.

The only reason mammography has become so entrenched is because mass cancer screenings – with follow-ups – is such big business. Out of 1,000 women, you have far more false positives than positives. That's not necessarily a bad thing for business because it leads to lucrative biopsies and other invasive surgical procedures.

On the other side of the coin, we have false negatives, that is, mammograms failing to detect cancer. In women aged 40 to 49, the rate of missed tumors is a whopping 40 percent, according to the National Cancer Institute. In women over 50, the false negative rate is 10 percent.

Incidence of breast cancer in Norway and Sweden during introduction of nationwide screening: prospective cohort study. BMJ 2004;328(7445):921-4.

[64] As reported in the Chicago Tribune, November 28, 2008. This was also in an accompanying editorial to Robert M. Kaplan, PhD; Franz Porzsolt, MD, PhD, The Natural History of Breast Cancer, Arch Intern Med. 2008;168(21):2302-2303.

[65] The Hope of Living Cancer Free, Francisco Contreras, M.D., page 104.

[66] This is the result of misinterpretation of Baye's rule using conditional probabilities instead of natural frequencies (in more familiar terms, relative instead of absolute numbers).

That radiation is harmful is without dispute. Just how harmful? Dr. John Gofman has made this startling statement about the impact of medical radiation:

> *"Our estimate is that about three-quarters of the current annual incidence of breast cancer...is being caused by ionizing radiation, primarily from medical sources."*[67]

Most people have remarked that Gofman's careful study must be an overestimate, but no one has ever shown how.

Radiation does two things: 1) It does physical damage to the body at the cellular level, which causes cells to mutate and become cancerous; 2) It weakens the production of white blood cells which constitute our immunological defense mechanism, the body's first line of defense against cancer.

Cumulative exposure to radiation from mammograms, in other words, can potentially do great harm. Not in the short term, but insidiously, years and decades down the road when it becomes very difficult to pin down the exact cause of a cancer. This is what J. Robert Hatherill has said on the subject:

> *"Women who received X-rays of the breast area as children have shown increased rates of breast cancer as adults. The first increase is reflected in women younger than thirty-five, who have early onset breast cancer. But for this exposed group, flourishing breast cancer rates continue for another forty years or longer."*[68]

Despite this, the American Cancer Society, together (of course) with the American College of Radiologists, has insisted on pursuing large-scale screening programs for breast cancer, including screening younger women, even though the National Cancer Institute and other experts are agreed that these are likely to cause more cancers than could possibly be detected.[69] In other words, aggressive screening may be replacing cancer deaths with diagnostic and treatment deaths.

This is borne out in the Canadian National Breast Screening Study (NBSS), the largest study of its kind involving some 50,000 women.[70] The findings: Deaths among women getting regular mammograms were significantly higher than in the group getting none. But here's the deadly twist: It was found that the mammograms themselves were not what was found to really accelerate the death

---

[67] Preventing Breast Cancer , John W. Gofman, M.D., Ph.D. See also, "The X-rays and Health Project. An educational project of the Committee for Nuclear Responsibility. www.x-raysandhealth.org.

[68] Eat To Beat Cancer, J. Robert Hatherill, page 132.

[69] The Politics Of Cancer by Samuel S Epstein MD, page 291.

[70] Canadian Medical Association Journal 147(10):1459-76 (1992). See also, A. Miller, et al. Canadian National Breast Screening Study: Breast cancer detection and death rates among women aged 40 to 49 years. Canadian Medical Association Journal 147(10):1459-76 (1992).

rate, but rather the conventional cancer treatments that followed! Precisely because conventional treatments are so toxic, they devastated their immune systems and killed the patients.

So, what is the take-home lesson? Mammograms are highly inaccurate; false positives lead to unnecessary tests and treatments; mammograms cause cancer; and when a cancer is detected, you are then subjected to treatments which can not only cause secondary cancers and other fatal diseases, but will severely weaken your immune system and accelerate your death. In other words, the real benefits of "early" screening go to the cancer industry, not the public.

So what should you do? You could try self-exams. Believe it or not, there is little practical difference in size between a tumor that can be detected by a mammogram and one that can be detected by self-examination. For self-detection, a tumor has to be around 1 centimeter in diameter (around half an inch), whereas a mammogram can detect a tumor at half this size. This is only one "doubling"[71] of the tumor and not a great difference that would affect the overall outcome of the disease in any significant way.

On the other hand, studies have shown there is little benefit to regular self-exams and good evidence of harm, including significant increases in the number of physician visits for the evaluation of benign breast lesions and significantly higher rates of benign biopsy results.[72]

There are a number of non-toxic screening methods, such as Thermography, 3D Ultrasound Tomography, as well as other methods currently being rolled out. Each method has its pros and cons, and the technology is rapidly developing, so you should investigate these on your own to see which might be suitable for you. The most important thing is to make sure you have a certified and experienced clinician doing the work.

But far and away, the best thing you can do to not only prevent, but fight, breast cancer is to follow the diet and lifestyle described later in this book. The benefits of doing that far outweigh anything else you can do.

---

[71] The 'doubling time' of a tumor is the time taken for the tumor to double in size. It's been estimated there are approximately 40 doublings between the development of a single malignant cell and the point at which a patient dies of widely metastatic breast cancer.

[72] Baxter N; Canadian Task Force on Preventive Health Care. Preventive health care, 2001 update: should women be routinely taught breast self-examination to screen for breast cancer? CMAJ. 2001 Jun 26;164(13):1837-46.

Five-Year "Cures"

"Cured yesterday of my disease, I died last night of my physician."
– Matthew Prior (17th century)

The five-year survival timeframe is an informative benchmark that has been used for years to measure the success of treatments. The perversity comes when the cancer industry starts saying that people are "cured" if they have survived five years following diagnosis. The cancer industry is the only part of medicine which uses such a preposterous definition because they're so desperate to show *any* success at all.

Whenever you hear a spokesperson for any part of the cancer industry talk about cure rates in the media, they are talking about five-year cure rates, not long-term cure rates. Good news is hard to find in the business of cancer, so they have to create their own. It's gotten so bad that lumps and bumps are now being classified as cancer even though they have not been diagnosed. And still others are classified as having cancers due to a bad diagnosis. In both cases, these "cancers" are entered into the books because patients survived for five years from a disease they never had. The really, really bad news is that they were also treated for a disease they never had.[73]

The five-year cure, aside from bringing in billions of dollars, is really what's behind the push for early screening. The earlier the cancer is detected, the greater the chances people will live for five years and thus be "cured."

This is what Dr. John Bailer, who spent 20 years on the staff of the U.S. National Cancer Institute and was editor of its journal, has said about five-year cures: [74]

> *"The five year cancer survival statistics of the American Cancer Society are very misleading. They now count things that are not cancer, and because we are able to diagnose at an earlier stage of the disease, patients falsely appear to live longer. Our whole cancer research in the past 20 years has been a failure. More people over 30 are dying from cancer than ever before... More women with mild or benign diseases are being included in statistics and reported as being 'cured'. When government officials point to survival figures and say they are winning the war against cancer they are using those survival rates improperly."*

---

[73] The Cancer Industry, Ralph Moss, 1996 Updated Ed., p. 29.
[74] Dr John Bailer, speaking at the Annual Meeting of the American Association for the Advancement of Science in May, 1985.

Most cancers are not found until people are dead because the cancers never caused any problems or symptoms. Thirty to forty times as many cases of thyroid, pancreatic and prostate cancers, for example, are found on autopsy than are ever presented to the doctor.

Prostate cancer usually begins growing in men in their twenties and steadily increases in incidence as they age. After age 70, about 80 percent of men have prostate cancer. This simply means that the immune system can hold these problems in check. But if the immune system is compromised by toxic treatments, all bets are off.

With prostate cancer so common, any excuse to screen and perform a biopsy is likely to find cancer in men over the age of 50, which means that scaring the patient into treatment is a sure bet. Even though prostate cancer occurs in most men, it has an extraordinarily small risk of killing them – only 226 per 100,000 in men older than 65. The problem is that if all men were screened and biopsied at this age, 80 percent would be told they have prostate cancer and would be treated. This means that 76,774 men would be treated for a disease that would never have killed them. Of the 226 men who would die from prostate cancer, the treatment itself has such a low success rate, it would not have helped them anyway – and in such advanced cases, the cancer has obviously spread beyond the reaches of surgery and radiation.

Thus, the cancer industry is now "curing" tens of thousands of prostate cases that would never have caused any problems were it not for the cancer industry's aggressive "screening for dollars" campaign and their relentless pursuit of the five-year "cure."

In other words, the increased survival rates are not the result of treatments, but a statistical trick.

As Scientific American observed some time ago, [75]

"The survival rate has therefore increased... because more men are being classified [earlier] as having prostate cancer."

The U.S. Preventive Services Task Force, The European Union Advisory Committee on Cancer Prevention, The Canadian Urological Association, American College of Preventive Medicine, The American College of Physicians and many others do not recommend screening for prostate cancer. [76] Why? It does

---

[75] John Cairns, The Treatment of Diseases and the War Against Cancer, Scientific American, Vol. 253, No. 5.

[76] Harris R . Screening for prostate cancer: an update of the evidence for the U.S. Preventive Services Task Force. Ann Intern Med. 2002 Dec 3;137(11):917-29; Advisory Committee on Cancer Prevention. Recommendations on cancer screening in the European Union. Eur J Cancer. 2000;36:1473-8; Ramsey EW. Early detection of prostate cancer. Recommendations from the Canadian Urological Association. Can J Oncol. 1994 Nov;4 Suppl 1:82-5; Ferrini R . American College of Preventive Medicine practice policy. Screening for prostate cancer in American men. Am J Prev Med. 1998

not reduce mortality and the treatments that follow devastate your body's ability to fight cancer, while degrading your quality of life.

The cancer industry will cite improvements in the five-year survival rate as justification for getting continued government funding. In 1970, for example, only half of those diagnosed with cancer survived to the five year mark, but today, decades and some $200 billion later, two-thirds survive. On the surface, this sounds like progress, but in fact, nothing has changed. People are simply diagnosed with cancer earlier and it *appears* as if they are living longer, whereas they are not. The natural history of the disease has not changed at all and the time of death is the same as it would have been had the disease been diagnosed later.

The five-year "cure" also serves to mask the delayed destructive effects of radiation and chemotherapy over time. The real terror of the five-year cure is that people live in fear that the cancer will return. Unfortunately, that fear is justified.

There was recently a story in the media that extolled new chemo treatments for early stage breast cancer, touting that 91 percent of the women were still alive after four years![77] Well, that sounds pretty breathtaking – until you realize that those women would have been alive without *any* treatment because breast cancer is a very slow-growing disease. Some accomplishment. And of the nine percent who did not make it to the four-year mark, the treatment itself, no doubt, accelerated their demise.

The Do Nothing Strategy

"Every really new idea looks crazy at first." – Alfred North Whitehead

"Time and time again it has been confirmed that the proven medical treatments are not only ineffective but dangerous. The vast majority of patients with cancer live longer and better if left without the orthodox treatments."
– Francisco Contreras, M.D.

"Most men with prostate cancer will die from other illnesses never knowing they had the problem." – Norman Zinner, M.D.

Jul;15(1):81-4; Coley CM. Early detection of prostate cancer. Part I: Prior probability and effectiveness of tests. The American College of Physicians. Ann Intern Med. 1997 Mar 1;126(5):394-406.

[77] Survival times increased significantly in early-stage breast cancer with Herceptin and chemotherapy, UCLA Health System Newsletter, 3/1/07; www.uclahealth.org/body.cfm?xyzpdqabc=0&id=502&action=detail&ref=322.

"I challenge anyone to show sound evidence that...advanced breast tumor patients do better...or even live longer, on surgery, deep X-ray, and chemotherapy, than they do when left totally untreated. In my experience, they don't." – Dick Richards, M.D.

"Most cancer patients in this country die of chemotherapy. Women with breast cancer are likely to die faster with chemo than without it." – Allen Levin, M.D.

"...the common [cancer] malignancies show a remarkably similar rate of demise, whether treated or untreated.... It is most likely that, in terms of life expectancy, the chance of survival is no better with than without treatment, and there is the possibility that treatment may make the survival time of cancer less." – Hardin Jones, M.D.

"I was contacted by a lady who successfully dealt with her breast cancer from 1994 to present. She refused all conventional medical procedures. Last year her conventional oncologist convinced her that she was a fool not to get a needle biopsy. This lady now has new tumors growing at each puncture site. Of course her oncologist now has detailed information to help decide which chemos to use for this now rapidly metastasizing cancer. I repeatedly make this same observation with prostate cancer. I rarely see distant metastasis until after a biopsy – and then it rapidly goes everywhere including the bones." – Vincent Gammill, M.D.

The "do nothing" strategy needs to be briefly discussed for two reasons: 1) It shows that doing nothing, medically speaking, is actually better than getting conventional treatments; and 2) You can and should take your time in order to research and explore the best treatment for you.

In the studies that have actually compared treated and untreated patients, they show that untreated patients live as long, if not longer, than treated patients do – and obviously with a higher quality of life.[78]

Consider what conventional treatments do to you. Chemotherapy not only destroys the immune system, the only thing that can ultimately cure cancer, but it can also destroy a person's stomach lining and the linings of their intestines to the point where a person's digestive tract can no longer absorb many of the nutrients in foods. This is one reason why many cancer patients die of malnutrition long before they die of cancer.[79] They die of nutrient starvation *as a result of treatment*. Chemo can also seriously damage every organ in your body. The toxins catch the blood cells in the act of dividing and cause blood poisoning.

---

[78] JAMA, 1992, 257, p. 2191; Lancet, 1991, August, p. 901; NEJM, 1986, May 8, p. 1226; NEJM, 1984, March, p. 737; Cancer, 1981, 47, p. 27; JAMA, 1979;241:489-494 ; A Report on Cancer, 1969, Hardin Jones.

[79] It's been estimated some 40 percent of cancer patients die of malnutrition.

The gastrointestinal system is thrown into convulsions causing nausea, diarrhea, loss of appetite, cramps, loss of hair and progressive weakness. Reproductive organs are affected, sometimes causing sterility. The brain becomes fatigued, eyesight and hearing are impaired and every conceivable function is disrupted with such agony that many patients elect to die of the cancer rather than to continue treatment. With bone marrow transplants, 20 percent will die from the treatment itself and a much higher percentage will die after the treatment. This is in spite of the fact that doctors will tell patients that the procedure has an 80 percent success rate (obviously a relative or "rubber" number).[80]

A study of breast cancer treatment with chemo said this:[81]

> *"Data on five-year survival [show] the benefit from adjuvant chemotherapy of breast cancer is only 4%.* **Mortality due to chemotherapy** *may be as high as 4.4%." (emphasis added)*

In other words, the therapy itself killed as many as it benefited. And the benefit was only four percent! Another study showed only a 6.3 percent 10-year survival benefit with those taking chemotherapy versus those who did not.[82]

I recently received a letter from a woman who had a friend with lung cancer. He was doing Ok with it, but once treatments started, he started rapidly deteriorating. It was clear the treatments were killing him and he died within a few months after the onset of treatment. It was apparent to her that he would have lived much longer without the treatments, and far longer with natural treatments – and with an obviously higher quality of life.

The following is a list of some of the side effects of conventional treatments:

[80] The 80 percent success rate for bone marrow/stem cell transplants is bandied about by doctors to patients as if it were really true. It is not true because it is a *relative* number. Meg Wolff, at the time a woman in her 40's, was given this fictitious success rate. (Becoming Whole, Meg Wolff, p. 63.) A friend recently underwent bone marrow transplant and was told by the doctor the treatment was "the cure" for his cancer. He bought the sales pitch and died six months later.

[81] Options, Richard Walters. See also H. Vorherr, "Adjuvant chemotherapy of breast cancer: Reality, hope, hazard?", Lancet (December 19/26, 1981), pages 1413-14.

[82] Early Breast Cancer Trialists' Collaborative Group, "Systemic treatment of early breast cancer by hormonal, cytotoxic, or immune therapy," Lancet 339(8785):71-85 (1992).

Abnormal ECGs	Gastrointestinal bleeding	Nausea
Abdominal cramps	Hair loss	Necrosis
Anemia	Hardening of veins	Neurological damage
Anorexia	Heart attack	Neuropathy
Arterial damage	Heart damage	Neutropenia
Arthralgia	Hemotologic problems	Nerve damage
Bleeding sores	Hypersensitivity reactions	Neuropathy
Bleeding ulcers	Hypotension	Numbness
Blood clotting	Immune system damage	Oral ulcers
Bone marrow suppression	Impaired concentration	Organ damage
Bone marrow destruction/failure	Impaired eyesight	Permanent disabilities
Brain shrinkage	Impaired hearing	Psychological distress
Cancers (secondary)	Impaired language skills	Radiation burns
Cancer cachexia	Impaired memory	Radiation poisoning
Chemo brain	Impaired thinking	Renal dysfunction
Chromosomal lesions	Impotence	Reproductive abnormalities
Chronic radiation enteritis	Increased infections	Sexual dysfunctions
Chronic radiation proctitis	Joint pain	Skin damage
Constipation	Kidney damage	Soreness of gums and throat
Cumulative toxicity	Leukopenia	Sterility
Cystitis	Liver fibrosis	Stroke
Deafness	Liver lesions	Sudden menopause
Decreased white cell count	Loss of appetite	Suicide
Dehydration (severe)	Loss of libido	Ulceration
Destroys lining of intestines	Loss of nerve function	Urinary bleeding
Destroys mucous membranes	Loss of taste	Vascular damage
Destroys skin	Lung damage	Vomiting (severe)
Diarrhea (severe)	Lymphedema	Weakness
Difficulty absorbing food	Malnutrition	Weight loss
Dizziness	Miscarriage	
Endometriosis	Myalgia	Toxic death
Flu symptoms	Nail thinning	

All clinics which use natural treatments will tell you that your chances of defeating cancer are far higher if you do not receive conventional treatments, simply because the treatments destroy the body's ability to heal itself of the disease. From their perspective, if you have conventional treatments, you will arrive at their facility as damaged goods.

According to a study by Dr. Ulrich Abel, 98 percent of patients treated with chemo die within seven years, 95 percent within five years. On the other hand, 98 percent of patients who do not receive chemo and receive natural treatments survive![83]

For those who have an aggressive form of cancer, they fail to benefit from treatment because the detection of cancer will be far too late to be of any help.

---

[83] As related by Dr. Ryke Geerd Hamer, founder of German New Medicine, referencing Dr. Ulrich Abel's article in The Lancet, 10 August 1991.

By the time an aggressive cancer has been detected, it has already spread throughout the body (metastasized) and conventional treatments are useless.

The sad fact is that after billions upon billions of dollars have been spent on research and treatment, people are not living longer because of conventional treatments. They are simply being given a longer death sentence. And due to early detection, conventional treatments are killing people sooner than if they had no treatment at all.

Here is what Hardin Jones said about the matter many decades ago and little has changed since then:[84]

> "My studies have proved conclusively that untreated cancer victims live up to four times longer than treated individuals. If one has cancer and opts to do nothing at all, he will live longer and feel better than if he undergoes radiation, chemotherapy or surgery, other than when used in immediate life-threatening situations."

My advice? Change your diet and lifestyle, but do nothing medically.

Saying Goodbye to the Cancer Industry

"To say that the new $10,000-a-month cancer drugs are a fraud would be an understatement. Even if you could afford to spend $120,000 a year to take these drugs, I'd advise you to avoid them. You'd think that cancer drugs that expensive would at least cure cancer, wouldn't you? But they don't! Half of all personal bankruptcies that occur in the US are due to medical bills and most of those are due to cancer treatments." – Randall Fitzgerald, The 100 Year Lie

"It's really exploiting the desperation of people with a life-threatening illness." – Marcia Angell, M.D., former editor of The New England Journal of Medicine, on whether the ultra-expensive new cancer drugs are worth the price.

"Patients who take every one of the high-tech drugs have to spend, on average, $250,000, suffer serious side effects, and gain, on average, [just] months of life." – New York Times, December 2005

"All told, the nation spent around $3 billion paying for it, while an estimated 4,000 to 9,000 women died not from their cancer but from the treatment." –Discover Magazine expose on bone marrow transplant surgery, August 2, 2002

---

[84]Transactions of the NewYork Academy of Medical Sciences, 1956, Vol. 6.

"Radiation and chemotherapy are crude treatments that will be obsolete before long." – Andrew Weil, M.D.

"In half the states in this country, it is illegal for even a medical doctor to prescribe anything other than chemo, radiation or surgery as a treatment for cancer!" – Jon Barron

In the beginning, the war on cancer was an earnest, if naïve, attempt to actually find a cure for cancer. Bolstered by the success of antibiotics and a landing on the moon, people were optimistic that with modern technology and enough money, anything could be accomplished, including a cure for cancer. Here are some typical sentiments, which are still being echoed today:

> *"We can look forward to something like a penicillin for cancer, and I hope within the next decade."*
> – Cornelius Rhoads, Sloan Kettering Cancer Center, 1953

> *"We are so close to a cure for cancer. We lack only the will and the kind of money...that went into putting a man on the moon."*
> – American Cancer Society full page ad in New York Times, 1969

> *"...with a billion dollars for ten years we could lick cancer."*
> – Testimony to Congress from the Director of the M.D. Anderson Hospital and Tumor Institute, 1969

> *"Cancer deaths can be cut in half by the year 2000."*
> – Peter Greenwald, M.D., The National Cancer Institute, 1989

> *"We are going to lick cancer by 2015."*
> – Congressman Benjamin Cardin, 2006

The cancer industry got plenty of money, but their focus on finding some "technology" that would cure cancer was totally misguided. Lost in the shuffle was the fact that a technology, or drug, does not cure anything. Only the body cures a disease. That basic fact was buried under billions of dollars of fruitless effort – and it is still buried today.

After some very limited success with chemotherapy and the treatment of obscure cancers, the years following the start of the war produced dismal results. Then, in the early 1960s, with the aid of federal legislation,[85] the drug companies

---

[85] One of the key pieces of legislation was the Kefauver-Harris amendments to the US Food, Drug and Cosmetic Act which declared that any drug, medicine, compound or device to be used in the alleviation or cure or cancer would be unlawful unless it is approved by the FDA.

took control and the once heroic efforts to find a cure turned the war into just another corporate play for profits. In fact, drug companies are in charge of your care, not doctors. If you want to know why there has been such phenomenal growth in cancer treatments, in the face of such failure to treat the disease, all you have to do is follow the money and look at the financial relationship between large cancer centers, such as the Memorial Sloan-Kettering Cancer Center, and the companies that make billions selling chemo drugs or radiation equipment.

> *"For decades, the war on cancer has been dominated by powerful groups of interlocking professional and financial interests, with the highly profitable drug development system at its hub."*
> – Samuel Epstein, M.D.

That cancer has become a major industry controlled by pharmaceutical companies leads to a series of problems. The first is that no one has an interest in preventing cancer because prevention does not produce big pay days.[86] There is obviously an interest in finding a "cure" because that's where the money and fame is; however, any cure must be proprietary (patentable) or no money can be made; and any cure must come from within the conventional medical community in order to justify all the money being raised and spent for research into a cure.[87]

---

[86] That prevention is an afterthought should be obvious if you look at the prevention budgets of any cancer organization. They are simply lip service.

[87] Most of the money raised for a 'cure' is ploughed into research that benefits pharmaceutical companies. That Big Pharma manipulates such fund-raising is illustrated by The National Breast Cancer Awareness Month (NBCAM), the brainchild of Imperial Chemical Industries (ICI), which became Zeneca Pharmaceuticals, and today is known as AstraZeneca, the maker of the breast cancer drug Tamoxifen. By sponsoring this event to the tune of millions of dollars, they are "pink washing" the fact this drug is ineffective and has significant side effects, including uterine cancer, liver cancer, heart disease, osteoporosis, depression, eye damage, blood clots, and even breast cancer – the very condition it is supposed to treat! AstraZeneca (ICI) is a chemical giant, and is one of the world's top producers of organochlorides, which are chlorine-based industrial chemicals, used in the manufacture of a wide variety of compounds, including Agent Orange, PCB's, and DDT. Organochlorides are also known carcinogens, and studies have found them to be specifically associated with increased incidence of breast cancer. So here we have a corporation – a very large and profitable corporation with billions in sales – that makes its money from 1) industrial chemicals that cause cancer and 2) drugs that treat (and potentially cause) cancer. Of course, you'll never hear anything about environmental causes of cancer from the NBCAM because AstraZeneca, being the sponsor, has the power to veto any materials which suggest links between chemical carcinogens and breast cancer. Thus, the main financial backer of NBCAM is a huge chemical company that makes a fortune off treating a disease they contribute to causing – and with a drug that has proven to be ineffective. Unfortunately, those involved in raising money for a cure are never told the truth – that pharmaceutical firms with deep pockets have convinced them to foot the bill for researching new drugs; that their money is being used

And while the pharmaceutical industry pulls the levers of the cancer industry, they, in turn, are controlled by the same gentlemen and women who run the major banks and corporations to which Big Pharma must answer.

In fact, the business of cancer is the second largest industry in the world and it is inextricably linked to the number one industry: petrochemicals. The ultimate decisions on what cancer treatments you will receive are made not in research hospitals, but in boardrooms of the major banks and corporations of this country. The next time you want to consult someone in the know about the newest cancer treatments, you might want to ask your banker, not your doctor.

Corporations have only one purpose in life: to make a profit. Corporations have a long history of breaking laws and causing death and destruction if the penalties for those deeds are less than the profits reaped from them.[88] Treating a disease such as cancer gives corporate medicine free rein: They can use deadly treatments without any penalty because death is so often the result of the disease. They are, in fact, getting away with medical murder. Cancer treatment is a corporation's dream come true and their profit will be at your expense, if you let them get away with it.

The longer the goodbye, the more profitable your cancer will be for the industry. The cancer industry will initiate the Cancer Cycle and push you down that slippery slope into pharmacologically plagued death.

In 1900, the risk of cancer was 1 in 30. In 1980, it was 1 in 5. In 1995, it was 1 in 3. Today, in 2008, after billions of dollars in research, your chance of dying from cancer are greater than 1 in 2.

In the year 2006, the cancer industry was delirious with self-congratulations upon learning that there was a decline of a mere 370 cancer deaths in the nation. The director of the National Cancer Institute, Andrew von Eschenbach, stated:

> *"It proves that our expectation of continued progress against cancer is well-founded."*

But as Ralph Moss[89] has pointed out, if progress continues at this rate, cancer deaths in the U.S. should be eliminated by the year 3508 – just a little more than 1,500 years from now.

In fact, the tiny dip in cancer deaths was the result of people changing their dietary and lifestyle habits on their own, not early detection or treatment. And such "continued progress" will come to a screeching halt as cancers growing in baby-boomers right now, raise their ugly heads and become detectable.

---

to subsidize research efforts of the wealthiest corporations which will turn around and charge patients hyper-inflated prices for patented drugs that don't have a snow ball's chance in hell of even approaching a cure for *any* cancer.

[88] See, for example, The Corporation: The Pathological Pursuit of Profit and Power, Joel Bakan.

[89] The Moss Reports Newsletter, February 19, 2006.

Modern medicine likes to trace its roots back to Hippocrates, who had a holistic view of the human body. The fact is, however, the roots of modern medicine rest firmly in the 17th century in which the universe – and later the body – were defined as a machine. According to this Newtonian view, the body could be analyzed, catalogued, adjusted and repaired as required, just like any other machine in an assembly line. Under this view, disease is no longer viewed as a state of the body, but a set of signs and symptoms which require management. Curing is the act of eliminating these signs and symptoms of a particular disorder. The underlying causes of the disorder, the conditions that support it, are irrelevant. A cure comes from a source outside of us, as we passively submit to a doctor's treatment and are "cured." The cure requires little or nothing from the patient and once cured, the person resumes his life as before and is largely the same person he was prior to becoming ill. Thus, doctors can prescribe cholesterol drugs to lower cholesterol and if the drugs lower it sufficiently, you are healthy again because that symptom of heart disease has been managed. You still have heart disease, but you are "cured." Similarly, chemo and radiation can push cancer under the radar until you are "cured." But you still have cancer.

To heal means to alter the internal conditions that created the illness in the first place and sustained its existence. Every serious illness – whether it's heart disease, cancer, diabetes, high blood pressure, digestive disorders or AIDS – arises because *conditions within the body* supported the birth of the illness and nurtured its life. To heal means to eliminate those conditions and replace them with conditions that support health.

When a doctor tells a patient there is no cure, it means that there is no treatment that the doctor can administer to eliminate the symptoms of the disease. It does not mean that the person cannot be healed. There is no cure for heart disease, for example, but we know that a person with heart disease can be fully healed and the illness eliminated from the body with a change in diet and lifestyle.

To heal, in other words, the patient must change his behavior and take charge of his health.

Note that the 'body as machine' paradigm works very well in many cases. If you break an arm, the doctor will work with that part of the machine and repair your arm. If you are wounded by a bullet, the doctor mechanically extracts the bullet, fixes the damaged area and you are once again healthy.

The problem with the mechanical approach is that is does not work at all with systemic diseases – diseases that manifest themselves as a result of a systematic failure, or degeneration, of the body. Yes, systemic diseases have symptoms, but treating the symptom is not going to correct the underlying systemic cause of the problem.

The beauty of dietary treatments is that they treat the body as a whole and work to re-balance a body that has become seriously out of balance.

This is what happens with all our chronic diseases. Adult-onset diabetes is a classic case of a body being out of balance. The American Diabetic Association says "there is no cure" for adult-onset diabetes and proceeds to recommend a life-long regimen of debilitating drugs, while giving lip-service to diet. But, in fact, Type II diabetes is cured quickly and easily for life with a change in diet. It's been proven time and time again,[90] can be easily replicated and yet, the top authorities of our medical profession continue to be the mouthpiece for drug companies and peddle their wares in exchange for donations drug companies give to their foundations.

The same act is being played out with our other chronic diseases, including heart disease – and cancer. This is not medicine. This is a white-collar corporate crime. And the sooner you learn this, the healthier you're going to be.

This book is not only about healing cancer, but healing the entire body. Because of the vast influence of pharmaceutical companies, we're used to thinking that we need a certain drug to treat liver disease, another drug to treat heart disease, and a myriad of drugs to treat the many degenerative diseases that are all caused by lousy diets. When you heal cancer with diet, the diet will also heal heart disease and any other degenerative disease you might have – all at the same time. In fact, *healing the entire body is the foundation on which a cancer reversal rests.*

A man was diagnosed with prostate cancer that had spread to the bone. A woman was diagnosed with breast cancer that had spread to her lungs. A man was diagnosed with kidney cancer that had entered his bones. Men and women were diagnosed with metastasized cancers of the ovary, colon, pancreas and liver. What did they all have in common? Their bodies were out of balance and producing cancer. What do they all have in common now? They got their bodies back into balance so it could fight the cancer, and they're all still alive, well and cancer-free. There are thousands of examples.

If your oncologist can't tell you what caused your cancer, how can he possibly treat it – and expect to cure it? The fact that your oncologist is not addressing the underlying cause of the cancer is the essence of what is wrong with the conventional approach to cancer. The fact he or she is only managing symptoms and is doing nothing to actually treat the cause of the cancer, is doing nothing to prevent the recurrence of cancer, is a telling lesson on how lost in the trees conventional treatment really is.

In fact, conventional medicine does not have a single treatment that addresses the cause of cancer and this is why it is completely helpless when the disease gains strength throughout the body, beyond the tumor location. The only thing known to mankind today that will stop cancer is for the body's own defense mechanisms to once again function normally. This is what nutrition therapy does.

---

[90] The vital facts regarding the relationship of diet to diabetes, and heart disease, as well, have been known for over 100 years and scientifically proven in the 1930s by Dr I. M. Rabinowitch and in the 1940s by Dr Lester Morrison. But they are still unknown to most doctors today.

It treats and heals the defense mechanisms of the body. And this is why nutritional therapies are so effective against cancer.

What, then, is the cause of cancer? The most experienced and knowledgeable doctors who treat cancers can answer this question in just a phrase: diet and lifestyle. And that means if you want to get rid of it forever, you have to make some big changes in your life.

If you are skeptical that nutrition and natural supplementation can reverse cancer, you should: 1) be even more skeptical that conventional treatments can do anything for cancer; and 2) be reminded that the entire medical professional was skeptical (and downright non-believing) when Nathan Pritikin totally reversed his heart disease by simply changing his diet. In fact, it took over 20 years and scores of scientific studies to prove that diet alone can reverse heart disease. Yet, over 40 years later, hospitals still do not employ diet to reverse heart disease. Why? There's simply too much money in conventional treatments.

The exact same thing can be said for the treatment of cancer. Just as bypass surgeries, stents, angioplasties and statin drugs all treat the symptoms of heart disease, without addressing what caused it, surgery, radiation and chemotherapy for cancer do the same thing. Just as arteries will clog up again after a bypass operation, cancer will return after the tumors are gone, precisely because the root cause of the disease has not been addressed.

When you come to realize that sulforaphane, a compound found in vegetables such as broccoli, Brussels sprouts and kale, actually blocks the growth of cancer cells, and that ellagic acid, found in berries, stops mitosis-cancer cell division, prevents the destruction of the p53 gene by cancer cells and causes cancer cells to commit suicide (apoptosis), to name just a few of the thousands of anti-cancer properties found in plant foods, you'll come to realize that there's something more to nutrition that meets the eye. There are thousands of phytochemicals in the plant food arsenal and each one works in symphony with others to effectively fight cancer, stimulate the immune system and put the brakes on cancer cell growth. We are just beginning to understand the powerful cancer-fighting tools in plant foods, but you don't have to understand a thing, other than what to put into your mouth.

You have no doubt read of studies which show that the consumption of fruits and vegetables do not lower the risks of cancer (much less reverse it!). One recent study involved The Women's Healthy Eating and Living (WHEL) Randomized Trial, of more than 3,000 women with breast cancer. The initial results? It found *no benefit* in eating more fruits and vegetables and less fat. The results of the study were published in the Journal of the American Medical Association (JAMA)[91] and headlines across the news read "No Cancer Benefit Found In Mega-Veggie-Diet Study," "Dietary Hopes Dashed for Breast Cancer

---

[91] Pierce, J. P. et al. Influence of a Diet Very High in Vegetables, Fruit, and Fiber and Low in Fat on Prognosis Following Treatment for Breast Cancer. JAMA 2007;298:289-298.

Patients," "Healthiest Diet Made Little Difference to Breast Cancer Survivors" and so on. And readers loved it because they could avoid eating that extra helping of vegetables!

What JAMA and the newspapers failed to mention was that the study was, in fact, fraudulent.[92] The women in the study simply lied about what they ate (which is not uncommon in survey studies). How do we know they were lying? Because their food diaries indicated the women, who were obese, were decreasing their average daily caloric intake by 181 calories a day over six years. That would have resulted in at least a 12 pound loss of weight – and yet they actually gained weight during the study! There are only two conclusions: They violated the laws of physics or they lied about what they were eating.

On top of that, their increase in fruit and vegetable consumption was extremely minor and the authors resorted to using relative (i.e., dishonest) numbers in order to exaggerate the increase in fruit and vegetable consumption, as well as the decrease in fat consumption. When put in absolute numbers, the differences were minimal, at best, and one would hardly call it a diet that could fight cancer. In fact, these poor women were eating the standard American diet, which *causes* cancer!

The fraud that was committed by the authors was to tell the public that cutting fat and increasing plant food consumption does not make a difference with cancer. There is a mountain of scientific evidence telling us otherwise.[93]

This is what Dr. John McDougall has said about the study:[94]

> *"I believe the authors intentionally deceived the public. One possible motivation for distorting the truth was to save face. They wasted $35 million dollars by feeding women with breast cancer an ineffective diet. Rather than admit their mistakes, they chose to distort the real meaning of the findings of their study, and effectually, deprive women of an opportunity to become healthier by eating more fruits and vegetables."*

The real tragedy is that an entire nation became aware of this study – that fruits and vegetables don't fight cancer – through headlines and only several thousand people know about its fraudulent nature.

Keep your skepticism intact, but keep your eyes open about so-called "scientific studies."[95]

---

[92] For an excellent analysis of this study, see The McDougall Newsletter, July 2007, Vol. 6, No.7.

[93] A very recent study, for example, showed that women who modestly increased their consumption of fruits and vegetables reduced their chances of recurring breast cancer by 47 percent. Marilyn L. Kwan, et al., Dietary Patterns and Breast Cancer Recurrence and Survival Among Women With Early-Stage Breast Cancer, Journal of Clinical Oncology, 10.1200/JCO.2008.19.4035.

[94] The McDougall Newsletter, July 2007, Vol. 6, No.7.

In general, the medical establishment – like all bureaucracies – is very slow to get the message, particularly a message that would require them to abandon treatments from which they make a living. It took, after all, over 200 years and hundreds of thousands of lives before the medical establishment began to accept the fact that vitamin C could cure scurvy – something "ignorant savages" had demonstrated to New World explorers in 1535.[96]

Despite the heroic-sounding "war on cancer" to "destroy the enemy" rhetoric, the body is not a battlefield, but a complex and sensitive system of self-regulation with profound healing possibilities. Your immune system is incredibly complex, easily rivaling your brain in terms of complexity, subtlety and self-awareness. And, yet, conventional treatments do everything they can to destroy this masterpiece!

Over 95 percent of all cancer patients who seek out nutritional treatments have already had extensive conventional cancer treatments and many of them had been sent home to die. Consider the condition of these patients when they seek alternative treatments:

1) Their immune system has been virtually destroyed by chemotherapy.
2) Because of poor immunity, their body is full of microbes and highly acidic.
3) Their cancer is stronger than ever as cancer cells have developed a resistance to chemotherapy.
4) Chemo has permanently damaged or impaired non-cancerous cells and organs. (A mortician can easily identify the body of a person who has been through chemo because their embalming fluids will not be absorbed by cells.)
5) At least one of their major organs (usually the liver) has been severely damaged.

---

[95] You can design a study to prove just about anything. Food industries have discovered that their propaganda goes down much better if it is disguised as a "scientific" study and this propaganda is published on a monthly basis. Sponsoring "scientific" studies is now a part of all food industry PR budgets. To the public – and press – it's difficult to tell the difference between a bona fide "scientific" study and one sponsored by corporate interests, such as the meat, dairy and sugar industries. Here are a few recent studies which sound "scientific" but are, in fact, pure propaganda from hired guns of food industries: Protein Metabolism in Response to Ingestion Pattern and Composition of Proteins (Journal of Nutrition, 2002); New Frontiers in Weight Management (Journal of the American College of Nutrition, 2002); Dietary Calcium and Dairy Modulation of Adiposity and Obesity Risk (Nutrition Reviews, 2004); "The Recommended Dietary Allowance of Protein: A Misunderstood Concept." (JAMA, 2008); Dietary Protein Intake Impacts Human Skeletal Muscle Protein Fractional Synthetic Rates After Endurance Exercise (American Journal of Physiology -- Endocrinology and Metabolism, 2005).
[96] America Indian Medicine, Virgil J. Vogel.

6) Their digestive tract is damaged and cannot absorb many of the nutrients from foods.
7) They are in extreme pain and, in many cases, have lost the will to live.

On top of all this, the window of opportunity for nutritional treatments has been largely lost – precious time that would have helped the patient rebuild their immune system so it could fight the cancer. The irony is that while patients usually turn to nutrition and alternative treatments as a last resort – after conventional treatments have failed – if a patient dies, the alternative treatment gets the blame!

If a patient starts nutritional treatments without receiving any conventional treatments, his or her odds of beating the disease increase dramatically. And this is the major reason you should say goodbye to the cancer industry.

In fact, there are thousands of biopsy-proven, advanced, medically incurable cases of cancer that have been completely reversed through nutritional therapy, which cannot be attributed to any conventional therapy the patient received.[97]

It's been found that those seeking alternative therapies are much more optimistic than those seeking conventional therapies. Why should this be so? Because they have only one worry – the cancer – not the cancer *and* the therapy.

If expensive, debilitating procedures to eliminate acne scars had the same failure rate as cancer treatments, they would have been abandoned long ago. It is only because cancer is so often fatal that conventional approaches have not been abandoned. We continue to use them not because they work, but the deadly nature of the disease disguises their ineffectiveness.

People like to ask, but will diet really help my type of cancer? It helps *all* types of cancer. Whether it is a carcinoma, a sarcoma, a melanoma, a lymphoma or leukemia, diet can be vital by helping rebuild your body's defenses. And if your immune system is healthy, it will know how to deal with every type of cancer. You should not be afraid of the type of cancer so much as afraid your immune system is not healthy enough to handle it.

Below is a short list of some of the cancers that have been healed naturally:[98]

---

[97] For 30 cases, see the book "Cancer Free: 30 Who Triumphed Over Cancer Naturally," East West Foundation, Ann Fawcett and Cynthia Smith. Critics say that cases in which patients received conventional treatments prior to nutritional treatment are not worthy of consideration because it could have been a delayed response to the treatment. Given the fact that conventional therapies are ludicrously ineffective makes this statement almost laughable. Of the cases in the book cited above, conventional therapy has not resulted in any cases of sustained regression or recovery from any of the cancers covered in the book.

[98] List compiled from various sources.

Adenocardinoma	Hodgkin's lymphoma	Oligodendroglioma
Adrenal gland	Hypopharynx	Omentum
Anaplastic astrocytoma	Kidney	Optic nerve
Anal canal	Large cell undiff.	Oral cavity
Anus	carcinoma	Osteoclastoma
Atrocytoma (low	Larynx	Osteosarcoma
grade)	Leukemia	Ovarian
Bladder	Liver	Pancreatic
Brain tumor (adult &	Lung	Pelvis
child)	Lymphoma	Peritoneum
Brain stem glioma	Lymphocytic leukemia	Pleura
Astrocytoma	Macroglob. of	PNET
Bile duct cancer	Waldestrom	(medulloblastoma)
Bone	Malignant fibrous	PNET out. nerv. sys.
Brain	histiocytoma	lymphoma
Breast	Malignant melanoma	Prostate
Bronchial alveolar	Malignant	Rectum
carcinoma	mesothelioma	Renal
Central nerv. sys.	Mantle zone lymphoma	Rhabdomyosarcoma
lymphoma	Mediastinal	Rhabdoid tumors cen.
Cervical	Melanoma	nerv. sys.
Choroid plexus	Meningiome	Sarcoma
neoplasm	Mesentery	Schwannoma
Chronic lymphocytic	Mesothelioma	Skin
Chronic myelogenous	Middle ear	Small cell carcinoma
Colon	Multiple myeloma	Small intestine
Craniopharyngioma	Mycosis fungoides-	Soft tissue sarcoma
Embryonal teratoma	Sezary synd.	Squamous cell
Ependymoma	Myeloid leukemia	carcinoma
Esophagus	Nasal cavity	Stomach
Eye and orbit	Neck	Teratoma
Gallbladder	Neuroblastoma	Testicular
Gastrointestinal tract	Neuroendocrine tumors	Thyroid
Germ cell tumor	Neurofibroma	Urethtral
Glioma	Non-Hodgkin's	Uterine
Glioblastoma	lymphoma	Ureter
multiform	Non-small cell	Vulva
Head	carcinoma	Wilms tumor
Heart	Nose	

If caught during the initiation or promotion stage, a true anti-cancer diet has a 100 percent chance of reversing the disease, in my opinion. Beyond that, the odds obviously become longer. When there is not complete recovery, nutritional treatments have extended patient's lives from months to years. In the worst cases, nutritional treatments have minimized or eliminated the pain and suffering patients endured in their final days. And in all cases, it has enhanced the quality of their lives, allowing them to spend their time living, instead of dying.

It's time you addressed the underlying cause of cancer. It's time to say goodbye to the cancer industry because they can do nothing for you, except take your money and damage your body. Only you can restore integrity and balance in your body. It's time to take control of your life.

PART 2 – Reversing Cancer

"Our way of life is related to our way of death."
– The Framingham Study, Harvard University

This book is about helping you reverse cancer. Conventional medicine classifies cancer reversals as mysterious "spontaneous regressions," and yet if you look into people who have made so-called "spontaneous" regressions, almost all had made major changes to a plant-based diet.[1]

According to conventional medicine, the rate of spontaneous regressions is so low it is essentially zero.[2] And, yet, we see cancer reversals all the time in treatment centers which use diet and lifestyle changes to reverse cancers. In other words, there are simply too many reversals going on in treatment centers to be either "mysterious" or "spontaneous."

Conventional doctors, including oncologists, have absolutely no experience with natural cancer reversals and think such reversals are extremely rare. But those doctors and practitioners who reverse cancers using natural methods know such reversals are exceedingly common – and there's nothing spontaneous or mysterious about them. This part of the book will help take the mystery out of reversing cancers.

---

[1] For example, see HD Foster, Lifestyle Influences on Cancer Regression, Int. J Biosoc Res, 10:1:17-20, 1988. See also the book "Cancer Free: 30 Who Triumphed Over Cancer Naturally", East West Foundation, Ann Fawcett and Cynthia Smith; Larsen SU, Rose C. Spontaneous remission of breast cancer. A literature review. Ugeskr Laeger. 1999 Jun 28;161(26):4001-4.

[2] When confronted with the evidence of natural cancer reversals, most doctors will go into denial, saying there was a delayed response to conventional treatment – despite the gross ineffectiveness of those treatments. When there was no previous treatment, they will say it was misdiagnosed and not cancer in the first place. When the cancer is proven by surgery or biopsy, they ultimately fall back on this spontaneous regression excuse – all because these cures do not fall within their medical understanding.

Rebuilding the Immune System

"Chemotherapy alone destroys the immune system beyond a point...which increases the risk for early death from infections and other cancers in these immunologically naked people." – Johan Bjorksten, M.D.

"I look upon cancer in the same way that I look upon heart disease, arthritis, high blood pressure, or even obesity, for that matter, in that by dramatically strengthening the body's immune system through diet, nutritional supplements, and exercise, the body can rid itself of the cancer, just as it does in other degenerative diseases. Consequently, I wouldn't have chemotherapy and radiation because I'm not interested in therapies that cripple the immune system, and, in my opinion, virtually ensure failure for the majority of cancer patients."
– Dr. Julian Whitaker, M.D.

The most important thing most people have to realize is not that we "get" cancer – because we get cancer every single day of our adult lives – but whether we "keep" and "grow" cancer due to: 1) a weakened immune system and 2) a body that allows cancer cells to thrive.

It's been estimated that at least 20 percent of Americans are clinically malnourished, with 70 percent being sub-clinically malnourished. What this means is that the vast majority of Americans are eating too much bad food and not enough good food. We're overfed, yet undernourished. Insofar as cancer is concerned, poor nutrition will impair your immune system. How can you tell if your immune system is impaired? A sure indication is if you catch colds, flues or other similar ailments. If your immune system is functioning properly, you should never, or very rarely, catch these illnesses.

If, because of poor eating habits, you contract a cold and eventually die of pneumonia, your diagnosis will be pneumonia, not malnutrition. And, chances are, your doctor will have treated you only for pneumonia, not malnutrition.[3] In other words, malnutrition is very common, yet hardly ever recognized as the reason behind an illness. The Western diet, which is so rich and seemingly varied, is in fact severely deficient in the foods that can prevent and reverse cancer. Malnourishment in Western countries is the result, primarily, of not getting enough *micronutrients* in the diet: the vitamins, minerals, phytochemicals and antioxidants that are so abundant in plant foods.

Each and every immune cell in your body is made from the food you eat and your army of immune cells will grow and become strong only if it has a good supply of micronutrients; and, conversely, it will weaken with a bad supply.

---

[3] Parenthetically, most doctors feed later-stage cancer patients garbage like Ensure®, which is malnutrition at its finest and a sure way to assist patients into their graves.

For years Japan had the highest per capita consumption of cigarettes, yet the lowest rate of lung cancer in the world, because Japanese smokers had strong immune systems due to their low-fat, plant-based diet.[4] Of course, now that the Japanese diet is becoming westernized, they are compromising their immune systems with a lousy diet and lung cancer is on the rise.

With respect to cancer, there are four "laws" that are irrefutable.

- Your immune system is the only cure for cancer.
- A weakened immune system is the biggest single cause of cancer.[5]
- The higher the dietary fat, the more the immune system is weakened.
- The only foods that contain significant immune-strengthening and cancer-fighting nutrients are plant foods.

Your eating habits can either strengthen or weaken your immune system. If you are not eating enough plant foods, you will be deficient in the micronutrients that feed your army of immune system cells. The goal of a good anti-cancer diet is to get the most micronutrients into your body, *per calorie*, that you can. An anti-cancer diet, in other words, is a *micronutrient-dense* diet.[6] The problem with all high-fat foods is that they are low in micronutrients, per calorie. You can only stuff so many calories into your tank, so the goal in fighting cancer is to get the

---

[4] Eat To Beat Cancer, J. Robert Hatherhill, p. 59. Of course, this hardly implies the Japanese have an ideal diet. Their high rates of stomach cancer have been blamed on the high sodium content of their diet. Corroborating evidence has recently been gathered by studies showing vegetable intake reduces the risks of smoking-related cancers. "Veg-eating smokers 'cheat illness", BBC News, 7/31/02; "Veggies cut smokers' cancer risk," MSNBC, 4/8/02; Protective effects of raw vegetables and fruit against lung cancer among smokers and ex-smokers: a case-control study in the Tokai area of Japan, C.M. Gao, K. Tajima, T. Kuroishi, et al, 1993, Japan J. Cancer Res. 84 (6): 594-600.

[5] Genetics accounts for only a small percentage of our common cancers. In the case of breast cancer, for example, genetics accounts for only 2-5% of all cases and this has been exaggerated. (See Part 3 - Genetics.) In terms of other external factors, it has been estimated that air and water pollution account for only 5%, alcohol and radiation account for 3% each, and medications account for only 2% of cancers. Diet and lifestyle factors account for the balance. For many individuals, genetics may make a contribution in subtle ways, e.g., it may determine one's susceptibility to carcinogens, the strength of the immune system, body weight and other factors. But each of these is also influenced by diet and lifestyle and such weaknesses can be offset by dietary habits, as illustrated in the Japanese smoker example. For more discussion on this topic, see Minamoto T, Mai M, Ronai Z. Environmental factors as regulators and effectors of multistep carcinogenesis. Carcinogenesis 1999;20(4):519-27; Cummings JH, Bingham SA. Diet and the prevention of cancer. BMJ 1998;317:1636-40.

[6] Although nutrient density is a popular term these days, it is sometimes used very loosely. The correct use is nutrient density *per calorie*. Many people have come up with their own way of measuring nutrient density, but the originator of the concept was William Harris, M.D., in his book The Scientific Basis of Vegetarianism.

biggest bang for your calorie buck. (See *Part 3 – Getting More Bang for the Buck*.)

The link between fat and cancer[7] has been observed by a former Surgeon General, who said that in comparing populations, "…death rates for cancers of the breast, colon, and prostate are directly proportional to estimated dietary fat

---

[7] Some examples: Calle EE, Rodriguez C, Walker-Thurmond K, Thun MJ. Overweight, Obesity, and Mortality from Cancer in a Prospectively Studied Cohort of U.S. Adults. NEJM 2003;348:1625-38; Cummings JH, Bingham SA. Diet and the prevention of cancer. BMJ 1998;317:1636-40; Chandra S, Chandra RK. Nutrition, immune response, and outcome. Progress in Food and Nutrition Science 1986;10:1-65; Barone J, Hebert JR, Reddy MM. Dietary fat and natural-killer cell activity. Am J Clin Nutr 1989;50:861-7; Hirayama T. Epidemiology of breast cancer with special reference to the role of diet. Prev Med 1978;7:173-95; Lands WEM, Hamazaki T, Yamazaki K, et al. Changing dietary patterns. Am J Clin Nutr 1990;51:991-3; Carroll KK, Braden LM. Dietary fat and mammary carcinogenesis. Nutrition and Cancer 1985;6:254-9; Rose DP, Boyar AP, Wynder EL. International comparisons of mortality rates for cancer of the breast, ovary, prostate, and colon, and per capita food consumption. Cancer 1986;58:2363-71; Rose DP, Boyar AP, Cohen C, Strong LE. Effect of a low-fat diet on hormone levels in women with cystic breast disease. 1. Serum steroids and gonadotropins. J Natl Cancer Inst 1987;78(4):623-6; Ingram DM, Bennett FC, Willcox D, de Klerk N. Effect of low-fat diet on female sex hormone levels. J Natl Cancer Inst 1987;79:1225-9; Goldin BR, Gorbach SL. Effect of diet on the plasma levels, metabolism and excretion of estrogens. Am J Clin Nutr 1988;48:787-90; Toniolo P, Riboli E, Protta F, Charrel M, Cappa AP. Calorie-providing nutrients and risk of breast cancer. J Natl Cancer Inst 1989;81:278; Hirayama T. Epidemiology of prostate cancer with special reference to the role of diet. Natl Cancer Inst Monogr 1979;53:149-54; Phillips RL. Role of lifestyle and dietary habits in risk of cancer among Seventh-day Adventists. Cancer Research 1975;35:3513-22; Mills P, Beeson WL, Phillips RL, Fraser GE. Cohort study of diet, lifestyle, and prostate cancer in Adventist men. Cancer 1989;64:598-604; Willett WC, Stampfer MJ, Colditz GA, Rosner BA, Speizer FE. Relation of meat, fat, and fiber intake to the risk of colon cancer in a prospective study among women. N Engl J Med 1990;323:1664-72; Gerhardsson de Verdier M, Hagman U, Peters RK, Steineck G, Overvik E. Meat, cooking methods, and colorectal cancer: a case-referrent study in Stockholm. Int J Cancer 1991;49:520-5; Singh PN, Fraser GE. Dietary risk factors for colon cancer in a low-risk population. Am J Epidemiol 1998;148(8):761-74; Giovannucci E, Rimm EB, Stampfer MJ, Colditz GA, Ascherio A, Willett WC. Intake of fat, meat, and fiber in relation to risk of colon cancer. Cancer Res 1994;54(9):2390-7; Gregorio DI, Emrich LJ, Graham S, Marshall JR, Nemoto T. Dietary fat consumption and survival among women with breast cancer. J Natl Cancer Inst 1985;75:37-41; Verreault R, Brisson J, Deschenes L, Naud F, Meyer F, Belanger L. Dietary fat in relation to prognostic indicators in breast cancer. J Natl Cancer Inst 1988;80:819-25; Newman SC, Miller AB, Howe CR. A study of the effect of weight and dietary fat on breast cancer survival time. Am J Epidemiol 1986;123:767-74; Holm LE, Callmer E, Hjalmar ML, Lidbrink E, Nilsson B, Skoog L. Dietary habits and prognostic factors in breast cancer. J Natl Cancer Inst 1989;81:1218-23; Donegan WL, Hartz AJ, Rimm AA. The association of body weight with recurrent cancer of the breast. Cancer 1978;41:1590-4; Schapira DV, Kumar NB, Lyman GH, Cox CE. Obesity and body fat distribution and breast cancer prognosis. Cancer 1991;67:523-8.

intakes."[8] In fact, researchers have recently called body fat a "highly active hormone pump"[9] which is constantly producing and secreting a wide variety of hormones, insulin and other growth factors into the bloodstream, as well as causing a multiplicity of other metabolic changes. The most dangerous fat is visceral fat, or the accumulated fat around your abdomen. In meticulously documented cases of terminal cancers being reversed naturally, there was a direct correlation between the reduction of visceral fat and tumor reduction.[10]

Many "experts" dispute the link between fat and cancer, citing studies in which dietary fat was cut from 40 percent to 30 percent and it had no effect on the incidence of breast cancer, for example. Of course it didn't! A 30 percent fat diet is a *high-fat* diet and *causes* cancer. You will not prevent the incidence of cancer until you cut dietary fat intake down to 10 percent of total calories – the same dietary fat level that reverses heart disease. Just "tweaking" the standard American diet has been the fundamental design flaw in Western dietary studies and such tweaking has lead to erroneous and disappointing results.[11] If you want diet to have a big impact on disease, you have to make big changes.

In every population throughout the world that eats a high-fat diet, cancer is the second leading killer, after cardiovascular disease. Among other things, high-fat diets suppress the immune system by killing off immune system cells. The higher your intake of fat, the lower your micronutrient intake and the more your immune system is weakened. Fat also reduces white cell production, which adversely affects T-cell and macrophage activity. And most tumors are promoted by high-fat diets.[12]

Imagine what an oil spill in the ocean does to the marine life it encounters. Most are killed, some are maimed. Birds covered with oil cannot fly. This is what happens when high amounts of fat hit your blood stream. Immune system cells die off, those that survive cannot "swim" in your blood stream, they become blinded, and as a result cannot recognize and kill cancer cells. Now imagine eating three high-fat meals a day. Americans have created a constant oil slick in their blood streams, caused by breakfast, lunch and dinner.

---

[8] U.S. Department of Health and Human Services. Surgeon General's Report on Nutrition and Health. DHHS Publ No. 88-50210, 1988.
[9] New Scientific Thinking Implicates Body Fat as Cancer Promoter, AICR Press Release, July 11, 2002.
[10] From conversations with Kushi Institute personnel regarding terminal cancer cases that were reversed with diet. For more information on these cases, see www.kushiinstitute.org/html/government.html.
[11] See, for example, The China Study by T. Colin Campbell and his critique of Harvard's on-going Nurses' Health Study.
[12] The genesis and growth of tumors: effects of a high-fat diet, Cancer Research Vol. 2, 1942, pp. 468-75; The role of follow-up and retrospective data analysis in alternative cancer management: the Gerson experience, Journal of Naturopathic Medicine, Vol. 6 No. 1, 1996, pp. 49-56.

You think I'm making this up? Take a look at the picture below.[13] It's a blood sample taken from a man who, hours earlier, had a cheeseburger and shake for lunch. The circle shows the fat content of the man's blood!

We currently have an epidemic of immune system impairment, which accounts for many of the diseases we are suffering from, especially cancers. In fact, we've become so used to a suppressed immune system we now think that getting colds, flues and cancers on a regular basis is normal.

Any kind of fat will compromise the immune system, even so-called "good fats" containing Omega-3 fatty acids. In addition to being an oil slick, it's been found that Omega-3's that come in concentrated forms, such as fish and vegetable oils, are composed of highly *unstable* molecules which decompose and unleash dangerous cancer-causing agents (free radicals) and cause damage to cells that can lead to cancer. Such fats also suppress natural killer cells and the production of immune substances, which are important for not only cancer protection, but also protection against viruses, bacteria and parasites.[14]

High concentrations of Omega-3's also promote the spread of cancer cells.[15] This is thought to be due to the production of free radicals, suppression of the immune system and changes that are caused in small hormones that promote tumor growth.[16] Unlike concentrated fats in fish and vegetable oils, the Omega-3's found in natural, whole foods are *stable* and do not produce free radicals. Thus, if you want Omega-3's, get them directly from whole plant foods, the original source of Omega-3's.

Eating concentrated sources of "good fat" really boils down to getting too much of a good thing. Just as a modest amount of sunlight can actually prevent cancer,[17] too much sunlight can cause cancer. Just as we need a little saturated fat in our diet, too much can clog up our plumbing. When vegetable oils are made, thousands of nutrients and fiber are removed and all that's left is 100 percent fat – or calories devoid of nutrients. This is an extremely concentrated form of fat

---

[13] Courtesy of Wellspring Media, Diet for a New America.

[14] Health implications of the n-3 fatty acids, Odeleye OE, Watson RR., Am J Clin Nutr 1991;53:177-8; Reply to O Odeleye and R Watson, Kinsella JE, Am J Clin Nutr 1991;53:178.

[15] Klieveri L, Fehres O, Griffini P, Van Noorden CJ, Frederiks WM. Promotion of colon cancer metastases in rat liver by fish oil diet is not due to reduced stroma formation. Clin Exp Metastasis. 2000;18(5):371-7.

[16] Effects of fish oil and corn oil diets on prostaglandin-dependent and myelopoiesis-associated immune suppressor mechanisms of mice bearing metastatic Lewis lung carcinoma tumors, Young MR, Cancer Res. 1989 Apr 15;49(8):1931-6; Influence of lipid diets on the number of metastases and ganglioside content of H59 variant tumors, Coulombe J, Clin Exp Metastasis. 1997 Jul;15(4):410-7.

[17] Cancer, January 2002;94:272-281; Cancer, March 2002; 94:1867-75.

and too much of a good thing, which will cause bad things to happen, like an oil slick in your blood.

Lowering the fat in your diet is the single best way to strengthen your immune system. Instead of a steady stream of fat, the RAVE Diet, described later, will lower your fat intake and provide you with a steady stream of cancer-fighting micronutrients that will feed your army of immune system cells and keep them strong.

Changing Your Soil

Louis Pasteur and Claude Bernard argued throughout their careers about whether the most important factor in disease was the condition of the "soil" – the human body – or, in contrast, the germ (which Pasteur was the first to identify). That is, whether germs are able to come into the body due to a weakened immune system or germs invade the body regardless of the state of the immune system. Bernard argued that germs could not exist in a healthy environment with a strong immune system. On his deathbed, Pasteur finally admitted that Bernard had been right, declaring, "The germ is nothing. It is the soil."

Conventional medicine has rejected the germ theory of disease, primarily because antibiotics were developed that were able to kill germs, regardless of the body's condition. While the effects of antibiotics can be dramatic and even life-saving, the condition and relevance of the body's immune system was lost in the glamour (and profits) of a very successful germ-killing drug.

In a similar fashion, conventional medicine believes that the tumor develops regardless of the condition of the immune system and then spreads to the rest of the body, much like an infection spreads with an army of germs. Others believe that the tumor is just a symptom of a systemic disease that is already present in a weakened body. The simple proof of how erroneous the conventional view is can be demonstrated by the fact that a detectable tumor has been growing for decades because of a weakened body. In fact, most cancers have a 10-to-20-year interval between their initial onset, or stimulus, and the appearance of a thriving tumor.[18]

A tumor simply means a colony of cancer cells has grown to be over a billion strong. Because our technology cannot detect the smaller colonies of cancer cells spread *throughout* the body does not mean there is no cancer in the body. Those colonies are merely under the radar. If you have a tumor, I can guarantee that you have many other cancer cells and colonies throughout your body that are too small to be detected. This is one of the sad misconceptions of our system: You only have cancer if it can be detected. Even worse, people are declared free of cancer just because it cannot be detected.

---

[18] Eat To Beat Cancer, J. Robert Hatherill, p. 23.

The real problem with this approach is what it means for treatment. The cancer is found in an isolated tumor and all one has to do is treat the tumor. Once the tumor is removed or destroyed, the patient is cured because the detectable cancer is gone. Much more important than removing the tumor, is removing the conditions in the "soil" that allowed the tumor to grow in the first place. Conventional medicine, of course, does not address this at all.

If you keep dumping sludge into a river, at some point you will meet a tipping point where the natural purification mechanisms of the river become overwhelmed and break down. If you simply stop dumping bad substances into it, eventually the levels of contaminants in the river will drop to a point where the natural healing mechanisms of the river will revive and clean the water.

Now, consider your body that river and consider all the sludge you've been putting into it for decades. Is it any wonder that cancer – and other diseases – has developed? Because of all the sludge in your body, a tipping point was created at some point and your immune system became weakened which, in turn, created a fertile soil for growing cancer cells.

Just like the chemistry of the lake, eating bad foods and leading a lousy lifestyle throws the entire biochemistry of your body off-balance. If you don't think changes in diet can radically – and quickly – change the biochemistry of your body, think how you feel after you've had a couple of glasses of alcohol – a little tipsy and buzzed – and all within just an hour. If you start bringing vegetables and other whole foods into your body, they will start to re-balance the biochemistry of your body and, over the long haul, make you feel much better than a couple of shots of booze.

In other words, it is just as important to stop bringing in the bad, as it is to start bringing in the good. It doesn't matter how many vegetables and other whole foods you consume, if you're still drinking booze, it will keep your body off-balance and nutritional therapy will be that much less effective.

If you can eat a bag of McDonald's fries without choking due to the high salt and oil content, I can guarantee the biochemistry of your body is sadly messed up because your body has become used to eating such trash.

Cancer is a degenerative disease. The conditions inside your body cause this degeneration and allow cancer cells to grow. Cancer cells are, in essence, a by-product of the deteriorating conditions inside your body. This is why the environment, or soil, is so important: It allows this by-product to grow.

A poor biochemistry can adversely affect healthy cells in many ways, one of which is to reduce their capacity to repair DNA. In a recent study of sisters,[19] it was found the sisters with breast cancer had a much lower DNA repair capacity than their cancer-free sisters. This resulted in a two- to three-fold increase in breast cancer risk due to the accumulation of DNA damage. Reduced DNA repair capacity is directly caused by diet (e.g., one component of DNA repair requires a

---

[19] Sarah L. Zielinski. Deficient DNA Repair Capacity Associated With Increased Risk of Breast Cancer. J. Natl. Cancer Inst. 2005 97: 81.

B vitamin called folic acid which is found in dark green leafy vegetables, fruits, peas and beans).

Here are four major conditions that cancer cells thrive on:

- High acidity
- Poor circulation and low nutrient/oxygen levels
- High blood sugar
- High cholesterol levels
- High sex hormones

High Acidity

Unlike normal healthy cells, cancer cells are able to flourish in a highly acidic environment. Conversely, they will not survive in a healthy, alkaline environment. The only way to change that environment? Diet.

Many dietary components can raise acidity, but the primary acidic component in our diet is animal foods, which are high in protein. Protein is made up of amino *acids*. This is one reason why high-protein diets are so strongly associated with cancer and low-protein diets are not. The vast majority of plant foods, on the other hand, are alkaline. Even lemon juice, which most people think of as acidic, is alkaline once it is in the blood stream. The ideal alkaline/acid ratio for our bodies has been estimated to be 80/20. Because of our dismal diet, heavy in animal (and refined) foods, this ratio has become out of sorts and far too acidic. In fact, the average American diet consists of only 20-30 percent alkaline foods and 70-80 percent acidic, whereas it should be just the opposite. And it's not all that unusual for the typical American to go up to two weeks without eating any alkaline foods at all!

The cells of the body in health are alkaline. In disease, they are acidic. The more acidic cells become, the less oxygen is available, the more stressed cells are and the sicker we feel and become. Our bodies produce acid as a by-product of normal metabolism and since we do not produce alkalinity, we must get it from foods to prevent our bodies from becoming too acidic. In other words, because our bodies are an alkaline entity, the majority of our diet must consist of alkaline foods.

Based on the USDA ash analysis of foods, here is a general chart showing which foods are acidic and which are alkaline.

Acidic	Alkaline
A few fruits & vegetables	Almost all fruits & vegetables
All animal foods	Raw nuts
Whole and refined grains	Sprouted grains
Sugar	
Herbs, spices, condiments, spicy foods	
Fried food, salt	
Sodas, coffee, tea, alcohol	
Drugs, medications, tobacco	

Throughout our history, humans ate a diet of primarily whole, natural – and alkaline – plant foods. Today, whole plant foods constitute *only seven percent of our diet!* 42 percent of our calories come from acidic animal foods and a whopping 51 percent of our calories come from acidic refined foods.[20]

Historical Percent of Calories		Current Percent of Calories	
Animal foods	5 percent[21]	Animal foods	42 percent
Refined foods	0 percent	Refined foods	51 percent
Whole plant foods	95 percent	Whole plant foods	7 percent

Is it any wonder that not only cancer, but other degenerative diseases are overtaking our bodies? In fact, it's been estimated that a whopping 70 to 85 percent of all hospital patients suffer from illnesses associated with diet-induced diseases.[22]

---

[20] Eat To Live, Joel Fuhrman, M.D., p. 51. In this estimate, oils constitute 11% of total calories. Oils are considered a refined food.

[21] Estimates vary somewhat, depending on the authority, but according to world-renowned paleontologist Dr. Richard Leakey, animal foods were a very rare part of the diet in human history. The five percent used here is obviously hypothetical, but may be even lower. [Dr. Richard Leakey, as quoted in The Power of Your Plate, Neal Barnard, M.D., p. 170.] When ancient man did eat meat, he probably walked, ran and jumped 20 miles to get it. And, aside from a very few areas where meat was plentiful, ancient man ate meat only a few times a year. In addition, the composition of wild game was a far cry from our grain-fed, domesticated, high-fat, hormone-laced meat that almost all Americans eat today. There were, of course, some populations late in our history that ate higher amounts of meat. They did, however, suffer the consequences. Autopsy studies of meat-eating specimens, such as the Iceman, have shown advanced stages of heart disease in 25 year olds. And that was from eating "clean" meat.

[22] Caldwell B. Esselstyn, M.D., as stated in the film Eating by Mike Anderson; The McDougall Program, John A. McDougall, M.D., p. 17.

Poor Circulation and Low Nutrient/Oxygen Levels

A second environmental component allowing cancer cells to thrive is poor circulation and low oxygen.[23] This is related to a number of factors, including high blood acidity. An acidic blood pH of 7.3, for example, has 69% less oxygen than an alkaline level of 7.45. Another reason for low oxygen levels is clogged blood vessels, the result of eating a lousy diet, particularly one high in saturated fats, which promotes blood clotting and lowers the delivery of oxygen to tissues and cells. This creates an inadequate flow of blood and immune activity. Because of clogged blood vessels, oxygen and nutrients cannot get into tissue areas and cellular waste cannot get out, which creates a cellular cesspool. This build-up of toxic waste can eventually lead to mutations and cancerous cells.

Unlike normal cells, cancer cells have adapted themselves so they can thrive without oxygen or in low-oxygenated environments.[24] A normal cell burns oxygen and glucose for energy and cleanly releases carbon dioxide and water. In contrast, a cancer cell produces energy by burning glucose (with no or little oxygen) and releasing lactic acid and carbon monoxide, instead of carbon dioxide. Back in the 1920s, Nobel Prize Winner Otto Warburg, found that cancer can thrive in a low-oxygen environment just like most bacteria. Every time he lowered the oxygen level by 35 percent in healthy cells, it consistently caused them to mutate and became cancerous.[25] The lack of oxygen in and of itself is not necessarily a determinant of cancer,[26] but rather creates an environment that cancer cells can adapt to and thrive in.

High Blood Sugar

This brings us to the third environmental component: *high* blood sugar (glucose). When you have high levels, you are feeding cancer cells because feeding on sugar is how they survive without oxygen. A recent study found that

---

[23] If you deprive a group of cells of vital oxygen, some will die, but others will manage to change their genetic software in order to survive. They will mutate so they can live without oxygen, deriving their energy needs from glucose and cellular metabolic waste products.

[24] One study has even found a significant association between a lack of oxygen in prostate cancer cells and the increased expression of the angiogenesis. See www.fccc.edu/news/2000/ASTRO-Hypoxia-VEGF-10-23-2000.html

[25] Otto Warburg, The Prime Cause and Prevention of Cancer, Revised lecture at the meeting of the Nobel-Laureates on June 30, 1966 at Lindau, Lake Constance, Germany. See also Otto Warburg. On the Origin of Cancer Cells. Science, vol 123, no. 3191, February 24, 1956.

[26] Oxygenation Therapy: Unproven Treatments for Cancer and AIDS. Saul Green. The Scientific Review of Alternative Medicine. Spring/Summer 1998, vol. 2, no. 1.

once blood sugar levels rose over 110 mg/dl, cancer incidence rose for leukemia and cancers of the esophagus, larynx, stomach, colon, rectum, liver, bile duct, pancreas, lung, prostate, kidney, bladder and brain; the higher the blood sugar level, the higher the incidence of cancer.[27] In laboratory experiments with animals, the tumor incidence for the group fed a high-sugar diet was twice that of the control group.[28]

Cancer cells consume 18 times more sugar than normal cells because they have more glucose receptors on the cell surface than healthy cells. The higher your blood sugar, the more you are feeding (and growing) the cancer. An oncologist friend was at a conference in Europe recently where there was a culture of cancer cells in a Petri dish. They added glucose to the culture and within 24 hours the cancer cells had doubled. PET scans are based on detecting "hot spots" where clusters of cancer cells are feeding on high levels of glucose. When blood glucose is kept at normal levels, cancer growth is slowed and the immune system is strengthened. Trying to beat cancer on a diet that raises blood sugar is like trying to put out a fire with gasoline. And yet, despite this, oncologists still offer candy to patients after chemo treatments.

In 1900, the average American consumed around five pounds of sugar. Today, the average American consumes over 140 pounds! That does not include the sugar that is consumed from eating refined foods such as standard breads, breakfast cereals, pasta, ketchup, canned goods and a myriad array of prepared or packaged foods. And drinking alcohol is the same thing as drinking sugar right out of the box, from your body's perspective.

One of the best things any cancer patient can do is severely limit or eliminate sweet foods from their diet, including sweet fruits. Fruits, by definition, are any food with a seed.[29] Thus, tomatoes, cucumbers and avocados are fruits, but they are not sweet fruits. Peaches, strawberries, etc., on the other hand, are sweet fruits. You can tell if they are sweet by simply tasting them. Yes, fruits have great anti-cancer nutrients, but vegetables, non-sweet fruits and whole grains do, too. You can easily limit or eliminate the sweet fruits and get all the cancer-fighting nutrients you need from other foods. The diet described in this book has a limited amount of sweet fruit in it because the goal is to starve cancer cells of their main food source, as much as possible. The goal is to keep your blood sugar level within the normal range and avoid blood sugar surges, which will feed the cancer. Once the cancer is under control, you can reintroduce sweet fruits to your diet.

---

[27] Sun Ha Jee; Heechoul Ohrr; Jae Woong Sull; Ji Eun Yun; Min Ji; Jonathan M. Samet, Fasting Serum Glucose Level and Cancer Risk in Korean Men and Women, JAMA. 2005;293:194-202. Before this study, it was difficult to disentangle whether it was diabetes or obesity that was contributing to cancer, but this study was done on a healthier and thinner population.
[28] Hoehn, SK, Nutrition and Cancer, Vol. 1, No. 3, p. 27.
[29] Technically speaking, if the seed comes from the reproductive part of the plant, it's a fruit. If the seed comes from the vegetative part of the plant, it's a vegetable.

High Cholesterol Levels

The only source of dietary cholesterol on the planet is animal foods and there has been a very long association between high cholesterol levels and high cancer rates.[30] There have also been studies which show that high cholesterol levels fuel cancer cells because cancer cells have higher demands for cholesterol than normal cells (similar to their sugar appetite). Growing cancer cells lose their capacity to synthesize cholesterol and become dependent upon outside sources, i.e., blood cholesterol. Studies have shown that by lowering cholesterol levels, it slowed tumor growth, reduced the spread of cancer and prolonged survival time.[31] In one study, a cholesterol-free diet cut tumor growth rates in half, compared to controls, and survival times were often doubled. When cholesterol was re-introduced into the diet, however, the tumors started to grow again.[32]

When animals injected with human prostate tumor cancer cells were fed high cholesterol diets, cholesterol was found to accumulate in the outer membranes of the tumor cells and altered the chemical signaling patterns within the cells. As a result, they resisted signals telling them to die normally and instead continued to proliferate in an uncontrolled fashion. While increased cholesterol levels did not trigger new cancers in the animals, six weeks after the tumor cells were injected, the animals on the high-cholesterol diets had twice as many tumors as animals on ordinary diets and their tumors were much larger. When their cholesterol was lowered, cancer cell death increased and the tumors stopped proliferating. When the cell membranes were replenished with cholesterol, it caused the cancer to run out of control again.[33] In other words, while not causing new cancers, high cholesterol levels were "feeding" existing cancers.

---

[30] Sidney S. Cholesterol, cancer, and public health policy. Am J Med. 1983 Sep;75(3):494-508.

[31] Cruse JP. Dietary cholesterol deprivation improves survival and reduces incidence of metastatic colon cancer in dimethylhydrazine-pretreated rats. Gut. 1982 Jul;23(7):594-9. See also, Chen HW. The role of cholesterol in malignancy. Prog Exp Tumor Res. 1978;22:275-316; Mady EA. Association between estradiol, estrogen receptors, total lipids, triglycerides, and cholesterol in patients with benign and malignant breast tumors. J Steroid Biochem Mol Biol. 2000 Dec 31;75(4-5):323-8.

[32] Littman ML. Effect of cholesterol-free, fat-free diet and hypocholesteremic agents on growth of transplantable animal tumors. Cancer Chemother Rep. 1966 Jan-Feb;50(1):25-45.

[33] Liyan Zhuang, Jayoung Kim, Rosalyn M. Adam, Keith R. Solomon, Michael R. Freeman. Cholesterol targeting alters lipid raft composition and cell survival in prostate cancer cells and xenografts. J. Clin. Invest. 115(4): 959-968 (2005).

A recent study made headlines (of course) by claiming that a low cholesterol level is somehow linked to (and may cause) cancer.[34] Nothing could be further from the truth! In fact, some cancers will *cause* low cholesterol levels simply because they impair the liver's ability to produce cholesterol. The people in the study who had very low cholesterol levels had undiagnosed cancers. Their low cholesterol levels were the result of their cancer, not the other way around.

High Sex Hormones

The last environmental variable concerns sex hormones. The higher these hormones are, the greater your chances of developing hormonal cancers, such as breast and prostate cancer (which are essentially the same disease[35]). From a dietary standpoint, high-fat foods (as well as body fat itself) are the main culprits raising sex hormones. Any time you take a bite into a hamburger, hot dog, chicken leg or any other high-fat meal, you're getting a hormone adjustment and altering the biochemistry of your body.

A young girl raised on a typical high-fat Western diet has much higher estrogen levels and, as a result, begins her menstrual cycle at a much younger age than one eating a plant-based diet.[36] In just 140 years, the average age of puberty in U.S. girls has dropped from 17 to 12 – and menopause starts four years later. In other words, women on high-fat diets have added nine years of menstrual cycles to their lives. How do we know diet causes this? Because women throughout the world, including those in the U.S., who are raised on low-fat, plant-based diets reach puberty at the normal age of 16 or 17.[37]

When women experience tenderness in their breasts each month, it's because estrogen is stimulating breast cells to divide and that's when a mutation, or cancer cell, is most likely to appear. If you have more menstrual cycles and more stimulation from high levels of estrogen, there's a much greater chance you'll develop not only breast cancer, but other hormone-related cancers.

---

[34] Yang X, WingYee S,Ko GT. Independent associations between low-density lipoprotein cholesterol and cancer among patients with type 2 diabetes mellitus. CMAJ 2008;179(5):427-437.

[35] Coffey DS.. Similarities of prostate and breast cancer: Evolution, diet, and estrogens. Urology. 2001 Apr;57(4 Suppl 1):31-8.

[36] Rodstrom, K. Menopause, October 2003; vol. 10: pp. 538-543, 2003; Am J Clin Nutr 54:805, 1991; Hum Biol 28:393, 1956; Int J Cancer 28:685, 1981; Nutr Res 7:471, 1987; Br J Cancer 55:681, 1987; Am J Epidemiol 138:217, 1993.

[37] When girls aged eight to ten increased their intake of vegetables, fruits, grains, and beans, and reduced their intake of animal-derived foods, the amount of estradiol (a principal estrogen) in their blood dropped by 30 percent compared to a group of girls who did not change their diets. Dorgan JF, et al. Diet and sex hormones in girls: findings from a randomized controlled clinical trial. J Natl Cancer Inst. 2003;95:132-141.

Milk is full of *bovine estrogen* from cows, so it's little wonder that dairy products have been strongly linked to breast and prostate cancer. Body fat also stimulates the production of estrogen, so the more body fat you have, the higher your estrogen levels will be. This is the reason overweight women have higher cancer risks.

Pesticides and other chemical toxins also raise estrogen levels because these chemicals mimic sex hormones once they are inside the body. Since 95 percent of the pesticides Americans consume come from meat and dairy products,[38] you're getting a double-boost to your hormone levels when you eat animal foods.

Breast cancer thrives in an estrogen-rich environment and estrogen levels for American women are up to twice as high as women around the world eating low-fat, plant-based diets. The problems American women experience with menopause is due to the *dramatic drop in estrogen levels*. If you get rid of this sharp drop, you get rid of the problems. By changing your diet before you reach menopause, the drop in estrogen levels will be small and smooth – and you will eliminate the problems. The Japanese, for example, don't even have a word for "hot flash" simply because Japanese women eating *traditional*, plant-based diets do not experience hot flashes – or other problems associated with menopause.

Eating a high-fiber diet is important because fiber removes excessive sex hormones from the body and lowers estrogen levels. If these hormones are not carried out by fiber, they are recycled back into the blood, which drives up hormone levels even further.

Men who eat high-fat diets also reach puberty earlier and have abnormally high levels of male sex hormones. Many studies have linked high testosterone levels to prostate cancer, but the most revealing fact is that prostate cancer simply does not occur in eunuchs, men castrated at an early age. Nor does it occur with men throughout the world who are eating traditional, plant-based diets, because they have normal levels of testosterone. Incidentally, you'll never see a bald eunuch because hair loss is also related to high testosterone levels. Although a tendency toward hair loss is genetic, you can significantly delay its onset and slow or arrest its spread by getting your testosterone level back to normal with a change in diet. In some cases, a change in diet has actually resulted in the re-growth of hair.

Eating animal foods stimulates the production of testosterone. Lowering those levels will prevent prostate cancer and slow the growth of any cancer that has already developed.[39] This knowledge has led to the development of testosterone-lowering drugs for the treatment of prostate cancer, but there's a simpler, cheaper

---

[38] Diet For a New America, John Robbins, p. 343.
[39] DePrimo SE. Prevention of prostate cancer. Hematol Oncol Clin North Am. 2001 Jun;15(3):445-57; Brawley OW. Prostate cancer prevention trials in the USA. Eur J Cancer. 2000 Jun;36(10):1312-5.

and more powerful way to lower testosterone levels: simply change to a low-fat, plant-based diet.[40]

Prostate reduction is also linked to a low-fat, plant-based diet and prostate cancer is rare in populations that eat such a diet.[41] Most prostate cancers have decades of slow growth before a tumor develops. This is the time when a change in diet can be most effective in strengthening your immune system and killing those cancer cells. And getting your testosterone level back to normal will not affect your manliness – only your chances of getting cancer – and perhaps going bald before your time.

Eating any farm animal today adds to your hormone overdose because large corporate farms use hormones to increase animal growth and output – and these hormones are passed on to us when we eat these animals or their products. Since 1995, Europe has banned the use of hormones in farm animals because of the links to human cancers. Europe has also banned American beef from its shores because of our continued use of hormones on livestock.

The modern cow produces 25 times more milk than a cow did just 50 years ago. A good part of that increased production is due to drugs, antibiotics – and artificial hormones. In fact, cow's milk turns out to be a hormonal delivery system as it contains over 50 different hormones. Numerous studies have shown links between the hormones in dairy products and the development of hormone-related cancers.

Imagine that you wanted to grow a colony of cancer cells in your body. What would be the perfect environment, at the cellular level? High acidity, low oxygen levels, high blood sugar levels and high levels of sex hormones. What would be the perfect diet to create such an environment? The standard American diet the vast majority of people are currently eating. I'm not talking about a junk food diet. I'm talking about the same diet most people think is healthy. And why shouldn't they? This same diet is promoted by government and university experts (who are under the influence of food lobbies pushing high-fat foods). This is same diet that is fundamentally altering the biochemistry of the body, weakening the immune system and creating a welcome environment that allows cancer cells to thrive. This is, in fact, the same diet that is causing an epidemic of cancer.

---

[40] Howie BJ. Dietary and hormonal interrelationships among vegetarian Seventh-Day Adventists and nonvegetarian men. Am J Clin Nutr. 1985 Jul;42(1):127-34; Key TJ. Testosterone, sex hormone-binding globulin, calculated free testosterone, and oestradiol in male vegans and omnivores. Br J Nutr. 1990 Jul;64(1):111-9; Habito RC. Postprandial changes in sex hormones after meals of different composition. Metabolism. 2001 May;50(5):505-11; Belanger A. Influence of diet on plasma steroids and sex hormone-binding globulin levels in adult men. J Steroid Biochem. 1989 Jun;32(6):829-33.

[41] When our common cancers appeared in traditional societies, such cancers invariably occurred among the wealthy classes, who could afford to eat rich, high-fat diets.

A healthy adult body has around 60 *trillion* cells and about a third of these make up our immune system. The essence of our bodies boils down to cells, intricately and automatically coordinating their activities so we can go on with our lives without having to worry about our health. Such a finely coordinated orchestration is truly a miracle.

Cellular activity is really the basis of all life and part of this miracle is that our cellular structure is able to repair itself when cells malfunction. Cellular malfunctions occur all the time. In fact, the average person gets anywhere from 1 to 10,000 cellular malfunctions in their body every single day. Chances are certain that you have cancer cells in your body as you read this and your immune system is (hopefully) already repairing the DNA damage.

The mechanisms in our body for repairing damaged cells are extremely efficient – until conditions inside our bodies begin to deteriorate and all hell breaks loose. Cancer, the disease, occurs when DNA damage is not repaired and cancerous cells starts reproducing themselves in an uncontrolled manner. These cells will travel throughout the body until they find an inviting spot where they will set up shop in a "bad neighborhood" of your body. If left unchecked, this bad neighborhood will continually expand until it becomes a detectable tumor.

Like the germ theory, whether we get sick or die has very little to do with what germ or cancer cell we get, but has everything to do with whether we keep our bodies free of the dead matter on which these germs feed – or clean up the environment in which cancer cells thrive. By changing the biochemistry of the body, we eliminate the conditions which allow cancer cells to exist. Once you do that, you won't need drugs to kill either germs or cancer cells.

Lowering Your Toxic Burden

Our bodies are exposed to an unprecedented number of toxins in our environment. The list of poisons includes pollutants, pesticides, carcinogens and hormones in our food, air, and water, electromagnetic radiation, tobacco smoke, antibiotics, prescription drugs, irradiated foods, nuclear radiation, mercury toxicity from dental fillings and seafood, X-rays, and the list goes on and on. Each of the toxins we encounter and absorb into our bodies makes a hit on our immune system and lowers our immunity.

The single most important thing for you to realize is that *the immune system is a limited resource*. Every hit to the immune system takes away resources that could be fighting disease, especially cancer. Avoiding and getting rid of toxins that are inside you is a sure way to lower your toxic burden and boost your immune system.

Pathologists are normally the only ones to do biopsies. But the sample should also be sent to a toxicologist, who can look for carcinogenic chemicals. In one case, a toxicologist found abnormally high levels of a variety of carcinogenic chemicals, including arsenic, DDT, DDE, PCB's and chlordane, as well as numerous pesticides and other environmental toxins. The patient was so overloaded with toxins, his liver could no longer detoxify his body and that created a welcome mat for cancer cells.

In 1973, a study by the Department of Occupational Health at Hebrew University-Hadassah Medical School in Jerusalem found that when cancerous breast tissue was compared with non-cancerous tissue from the same woman's body, the concentration of toxic chemicals, such as DDT and PCBs, was "much increased in the malignant tissue compared to the normal breast and adjacent adipose tissue."[42]

Because of this study, Israel banned these chemicals from feed for dairy cows and cattle. Over the next ten years, the rate of breast cancer deaths in Israel declined sharply. The only answer scientists could find to explain this was the reduced level of environmental toxins.

We spray 1.2 billion pounds of pesticides on (non-organic) produce every year, there are now over 2,800 FDA-approved food additives in our food, and we feed over five million pounds of antibiotics every year to farm animals to make them grow faster. The EPA estimates that 40 percent of U.S. fresh water is unusable and there are 1,300 different chemicals in the average EPA-approved city drinking water. There are 60,000 chemicals in regular use, half of these in direct contact with humans. We have found residues of the lethal industrial solvent PCB and the pesticide DDT in every human on earth – as well as in mother's milk.

In other words, our bodies are very contaminated and that contamination is causing cancers in some people. I say in "some" people because with the proper diet and lifestyle, our bodies are more than capable of ridding themselves of toxins, even at these high levels.

Some simple steps you can take to lower your toxic burden would be to avoid all known or possible carcinogenic substances you might come across, as best you can. This would include environmental carcinogens, microwaves and micro-waved food, food and water stored in plastic containers (use glass or ceramic), as well as synthetic clothing, bedding and carpets (due to the chemicals used in synthetics). Stick to natural fibers and replace your carpet with wood flooring, if you can afford to (it's actually cheaper in the long run). Also invest in a good water filter for both drinking and showering.

The single best way to avoid dietary toxins is to eat certified organic plant foods.

Another step you can take to detoxify your body is to avoid all prescription drugs. Prescription drugs – without exception – are toxic to the body and all have side effects. The most common cause of side effects is the simple fact that

---

[42] Congress of the United States House of Representatives Committee on Government Reform Hearing on "Integrative Oncology - Cancer Care for the New Millennium" June 7 and 8, 2000 Washington, D.C., Testimony of Burton Goldberg.

prescription drugs are highly concentrated and not found in nature, so they're hard on the liver. Once your liver is chronically stressed by taking a drug every day, any additional stress you put on it, such as exposure to everyday toxins (e.g., car exhaust, paint fumes, pesticides, excess alcohol, etc.) can compromise your health because it will increase the level of toxins in your body. The liver is crucial to detoxifying your body and strengthening your immune system. Prescription drugs will prevent that detoxification.

If you are taking drugs for a chronic, degenerative disease, a true anti-cancer diet will also heal those diseases while it fights cancer, so you can wean yourself off the drugs as your condition improves. Work with your physician on this and tell him or her about your change in diet. If your physician does not support your change in diet, get one who does. If you do not know of one, consult www.RaveDiet.com, which has a list of doctors and clinics which practice nutritional therapy.

Colon Cleansing

Many clinics employ colon cleansing as a way to clean out your body and accelerate the detoxification process. Many people's colons are packed with a lifetime of old, hardened feces, which leads to the accumulation of poisons. During one colon cleanse, half of a crayon came out of a 70-year-old man – a crayon the man had swallowed as a child! The build-up of toxic material in your colon takes away resources from your immune system because the immune system is continually fighting this self-poisoning. By cleaning out the colon, you free-up immune system resources.

In addition, one of the colon's main functions is to absorb the nutrients our body needs through its walls. If there is a layer of toxic sludge on the walls, vitamins, minerals, enzymes and other nutrients cannot pass through the hardened walls of the colon. When this sludge is removed, the body will again begin to utilize nutrients from foods.

Dr. Harvey Kellogg, of the Kellogg Sanitarium in Battle Creek Michigan, said this about colons:[43]

> "Of the 22,000 operations that I have personally performed, I have never found a single normal colon. Of the 100,000 that were performed under my jurisdiction, not over 6% were normal."

One expert on the subject estimates that the average 35-year-old has four to 22 pounds of undigested sludge in their intestine, even according to the FDA.[44] A

---

[43] Quoted in Journey to the Center of Your Colon, Tim O'Shea. See www.thedoctorwithin.com/colon/Journey-to-the-Center-of-Your-Colon.php

[44] Cleanse and Purify, Richard Anderson.

chiropractor who writes extensively on the subject has said that on autopsy, John Wayne had 44 pounds of toxic sludge build-up, while Elvis had 22 pounds.[45] If you think this is an exaggeration, search on the web for the phrase "mucoid plaque" and look at the pictures. Here's one example:[46]

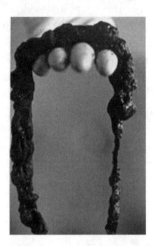

As a first step in the detoxification of your body, I would recommend a colon cleanse. You can find a Colon Hydrotherapist near you by visiting the Resources section at www.RaveDiet.com. Colonics are not enemas and they require a professional with professional equipment to administer them. Once your colon is cleaned, the RAVE Diet will keep it clean.

There are other organ-cleansing steps you can take and your Colon Hydrotherapist can tell you about these. Without question, however, the colon cleanse is the most important.

---

[45] Enzymes: The Key to Longevity, Tim O'Shea. This can be found at: www.thedoctorwithin.com/enzymes/Enzymes-The-Key-to-Longevity.php.
[46] Courtesy of www.detox-cleanse.com/images/mucoid-plaque.jpg.

Attitude

"Every cell in your body is eavesdropping on your thoughts."
– Deepak Chopra, M.D.

If we could find a way to harness the power of the mind and direct it toward healing illnesses, we could live disease-free for the rest of our lives. The mind can be that powerful.

The problem, of course, is that for the vast majority of humans, the mind does not overtly come into play at all with the body. If it did, we would hear more about it. Many more positive outcomes would be observed among people who join self-healing groups, pray or visit Lourdes. Unfortunately, despite intense interest in such mind-body cures over the millennia – whether religious or secular, scientific or mystical – none of the approaches based on mind or spirit have proven to be particularly effective. Even the famed Lourdes, with over a million visitors a year, boasts of only a few dozen "miracle cures" – ever.

This is not to say the mind cannot play a role in heath, but we should talk about states of the mind, not miracles, because although the mind and body communicate constantly with each other, most of this communication is on an unconscious level and largely beyond our direct control.

Although the influence of the mind can be profound, the healing power of the mind will vary from individual to individual. And it should not be relied on to produce a cure. If anything, it should be regarded as a "supplement," not the main treatment simply because the odds are very long against it working to heal an illness.

If you had two groups of people and one group relied on the mind (or spirit), while the other group relied on a good cancer-fighting diet, the nutritional group would win easily – reliably and consistently. While the mind can be a healer for some people, proper nutrition is the key to consistent success.

As a practical matter, attitude is important with respect to treatment because the patient must be behind the treatment, thinking that it will work. Positive thinking can have an effect in helping push the treatment along, just like a supplement. In my opinion, positive thinking is so important that if a patient truly believes that conventional therapy will work for them and nutrition therapy will not, I would tell them to stick to their conventional therapy. A sour attitude, in other words, can spoil the treatment pot.

An angry, stressed or depressed mind can suppress the immune system and allow cancer to grow. In one study, it was found that depression doubled the risk of cancer. We know that some people who are under severe temporary stress make more cancer cells than usual. And once they feel better, the clusters of cancerous cells disappear. What happens is that secretions of the DNA's anti-cancer drug, Interleukin II, are lowered under physical and mental duress and increase again when relaxed and joyful.

Controlled clinical trials have shown that some 30 to 40 percent of depressed patients who are given placeboes get better – a treatment effect that antidepressants barely top.[47] Of course, the placebo effect has to do with expectations. If you expect something to happen, your brain will help make it happen. Therein lies the magic of positive thinking. Just as patients on chemotherapy throw up *on the way* to their oncologist's office due to their expectation of what will happen there, patients who were given a chemotherapy placebo have had their hair fall out![48]

Advertisers have known about expectations for years and studies have shown that more expensive fake medicines work much better than cheap fake medicines. People often think generic medicine is inferior, but gussy it up a bit, change the name, make it appear more expensive and the same fake medicine will actually work better!

Previously, I stated that the mind should be considered a "supplement" and in that regard, the major ingredient in this supplement should be laughter, because it stimulates the immune system like nothing else in the world.[49] Norman Cousins, who was fighting an "incurable" degenerative disease, trained himself to belly laugh by watching comedies like the *Marx Brothers* and *Candid Camera*.[50] As he put it:

> *"I made the joyous discovery that ten minutes of genuine belly laughter had an anesthetic effect and would give me at least two hours of pain-free sleep. When the pain-killing effect of the laughter wore off, we would switch on the motion picture projector again and not infrequently, it would lead to another pain-free interval."*

He checked himself out of the hospital and began a remarkable journey of self-healing by giving himself an attitude adjustment.

The bottom line: Your expectations about healing cancer should be optimistic, but realistic, because just as placebos can be successful, expectations have a way of becoming self-fulfilling. You should always anticipate recovery instead of further illness. You should always listen to your hopes, not your fears and always feel in control, never helpless. A refusal to hope is nothing more than a decision to die because there are no incurable diseases, only incurable people.

---

[47] Half of Doctors Routinely Prescribe Placebos, NY Times, 10/22/08.

[48] This reference is from the film, When Healing Becomes a Crime by Kenny Ausubel when interviewing Bernie Siegel, M.D. It is also mentioned in Love, Medicine and Miracles by Bernie Siegel, M.D., p. 133, where a group of men were given saline and told it was chemotherapy. Thirty percent had their hair fall out.

[49] For those interested in the relationship between the mind and immune system, look up Psychoneuroimmunology, which is the branch of science devoted to this topic.

[50] The Anatomy of an Illness, Norman Cousins.

Visualization

A very simple, yet powerful, trick will help keep you on the course you have chosen. What you should do is relax, breath evenly, close your eyes and visualize what you will look like once the cancer is gone and you have adopted a new lifestyle. Picture yourself walking, running and playing. Picture what you will look like in new clothes, at social occasions and in every different situation you can imagine in your new lifestyle. Visualize everything that you associate with your new lifestyle – a new attitude, confidence, new friends and so forth. No doubt, it is a very happy sight.

Spend a few minutes running these visualizations through your mind, then lock in the images. Do this frequently. You simply can't do it too often.

Every time you have a bad feeling, take a deep breath, close your eyes and run those images through your mind.

Some people make "vision boards" where they cut out pictures from magazines and newspapers and paste them onto a board. It ends up as a collage of images representing what their lifestyle goals are. After they have finished their collage, they hang it up in a place so they will see it every single day to remind them of what they are striving for.

There are an infinite number of variations to this theme. It's simply asserting mind over body in order to get you where you want your body to be. Always keep the positive images in your head. They will steer you in the right direction and keep you moving forward toward your new lifestyle.

The Pursuit of Happiness

"The goal in life is to die young – as late as possible." – Ashley Montagu

The relationship between diet and disease is as old as the Bible. You may recall the biblical story of Daniel. After suffering through ill health, Daniel made a radical proposal to take the servants off their rich, royal diet and put them on a diet of vegetables and water. In only ten days, the servants looked healthier and better nourished than any of the other men who had eaten the royal foods.

You don't have to eat just vegetables and water to achieve the health of Daniel's servants and the remainder of this book shows you how to eat a wide variety of delicious, natural foods that will truly do wonders for your body.

Our bodies are incredibly smart. We have *trillions* of cells intricately and automatically coordinating their activities so we can go on with our lives without having to worry about our health. But when we introduce bad foods to our bodies, we start to destroy this finely tuned masterpiece, balance is lost and the preconditions for disease set in. Our bodies scramble to recover and regain balance, but so long as bad food keeps coming in, the body will remain out of balance and, over time, disease will take over. Our bodies are extremely forgiving of bad habits – but only up to a point – and when they have had enough, we'll get a wakeup call like the one we've never had before.

One of the most brilliant passages ever written is in the U.S. Constitution when the writers declared the pursuit of happiness to be an "unalienable right." For me, the measure of a good life is how much happiness you get out of it. To me, the pursuit of happiness is really about owning *less* stuff, while gaining *more* purpose in life. "Stuff" brings temporary pleasure. Purpose brings lasting pleasure. People who look outside of themselves for happiness by pursuing "stuff" are always disappointed because long-term happiness inevitably springs from within. The same can be said for your health. Health *always* comes before wealth and you must remind yourself of that when setting your priorities.

Depression is the consequence of seeking excessive stimulation. When you strive to experience extreme "highs," you will inevitably end up depressed when the exhilaration from those highs wears off. Always seek to find your middle ground. Balance your life. Seek purpose in it and go for more than just the temporary, immediate highs which life has to offer.

For every immediate pleasure you give up, you gain something more valuable and lasting. The smoker or alcoholic who gives up his destructive habit gains much more than he loses. You will gain much more by giving up the "pleasure traps" of our standard destructive diet. I've seen people transformed by the RAVE Diet. I've seen men, who used to grill steaks on the barbeque during football games, now talking about the best way to make chopped salad.

Dare to be different. Change your life and seek long-term happiness from within by adopting a lifestyle that I guarantee will pay countless dividends throughout your entire life.

PART 3 – The RAVE Diet & Lifestyle

"Nature distributed medicine everywhere." – Pliny the Elder, A.D. 77

"Natural forces within us are the true healers." – Hippocrates

"The ideal of medicine is to eliminate the need of a physician."
– William J. Mayo, founder of the Mayo Clinic

"Eating a plant-based diet all year long is the best way to help lower your risk of cancer." – The Dana-Farber Cancer Institute

There is a very long history of reversing cancer with diets, ranging from macrobiotic to raw diets and several in-between, including the RAVE Diet. What do all these diets have in common? They are plant-based. In fact, you cannot find a clinic with a strong track record of reversing cancer using animal-based diets. And the most successful of these clinics use 100 percent plant-based diets. The other thing these diets have in common is a *complete and total* switch to the diet. Your goal is to change the biochemistry of your body in order to make it hostile to cancer and nothing less than a complete and consistent change in diet will do that.

So-called "super foods" are in the news right now. For example, "A cup of black tea each day reduces risk of Parkinson's disease by an astonishing 71 percent;" vitamin D reduces the risk of cancer by 70 percent; blueberries fight this type of cancer; curry fights that type of cancer; a chemical in raspberries causes certain cancer cells to commit suicide. And so forth. But if you're eating burgers and cheesecake every day, it won't matter how many cups of tea you drink. You can choke on blueberries but it won't make any difference if the rest of your diet is in the toilet. It's not this "superfood" or that "superfood," but your *overall dietary profile* that matters.

There have been a number of studies that show when a single cancer-preventive nutrient was fed to animals it had no effect on the incidence of cancer. But when two or more nutrients were combined, the cancer growth was sharply cut.[1]

In a similar fashion, supplements provide only limited benefits since they usually contain only one specific, *isolated* phytochemical or antioxidant. Vitamin E only fights a specific type of free radical, but when combined with other antioxidants (e.g., beta carotene, lycopene and flavonoids) the benefits are far

---

[1] Rao, AR, et al. Japanese J. Cancer Research. vol. 81, p. 1239; Jo, J. Journal of Agricultural and Food Chemistry, April 6, 2005; vol 53: pp 2489-2498.

greater than the benefits of vitamin E taken alone. This is because of the synergistic, cooperative interaction between antioxidants.[2]

Conversely, it's been found that when blueberries are consumed with milk, the activity of antioxidants is greatly reduced.[3] And it's not just milk, but any high-protein food. In other words, all the foods comprising your dietary profile have to be pointing in the same direction. This is what the RAVE Diet does for you.

What these studies examined were just a few nutrients, not the thousands and thousands of combinations that go on inside your body every day in the real world. When you're eating a diet low in plant nutrients (and there are over 25,000 nutrients from plants that are rich in *cancer*-fighting phytochemicals), your body doesn't have a chance to experience the logarithmic power of these foods working together in the same direction to fight cancer.

The point is this: when scientists try to isolate a single nutrient or even a handful of nutrients in a food and call it a "superfood," this is far too simplistic. The single or multiple nutrient analysis is like the six blind men trying to 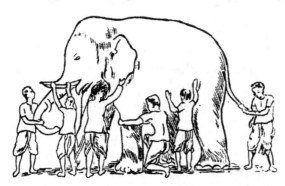 understand the nature of an elephant: They will never understand what the whole elephant is, but only selected parts of it. While science will continue to identify key nutrients in foods, it is a certainty that science will never understand how the millions of nutrients interact with each other as a whole. The mathematical possibilities are simply too immense.

There is, in other words, "magic" in whole plant foods and we do not comprehend how this magic works. What we do know is that we should eat a wide variety of plant foods because each food has its own nutrient profile, it will interact with other plant foods containing their own profile and, together, they will amplify each other's benefits in a logarithmic fashion.

One of the most common themes in letters I receive is that people claimed to have been eating a healthy diet, did not drink or smoke, jogged at least four times a week and participated in yoga classes at least twice a week – and yet still got cancer. The lifestyle choices they made were all good but always, upon closer examination, their "healthy" diet was far from healthy and did not have a chance

---

[2] Bianca Fuhrman, et al. Lycopene Synergistically Inhibits LDL Oxidation in Combination with Vitamin E, Glabridin, Rosmarinic Acid, Carnosic Acid, or Garlic. Antioxidants & Redox Signaling. September 2000: 491-506.
[3] Mauro Serafinia, et al. Antioxidant activity of blueberry fruit is impaired by association with milk. Free Radical Biology and Medicine. (online) 11 December 2008.

to prevent cancer. Once we get into the RAVE Diet, you will see how far removed it is from your typical "healthy" diet. The diet is strict, some may say "radical," and yet it is delicious and quite easy to follow once you try it. And if you want a chance at reversing the cancer, you will have to become the Mother Teresa of nutrition. Once the cancer is under control, however, you can relax a little, but not much. This diet is designed to keep you healthy and fit for the rest of your life and if you follow it closely, the dividends will be immense.

The RAVE Diet is not about restricting food portions, but *changing food choices* and breaking through the vicious eating cycles that are making people sick. Without a doubt, it will be more difficult for some than others. We're talking about re-training your taste buds, which usually takes about three weeks. The problem is that we've lost our taste for natural foods because most of the food we eat today is smothered with salt, fat, sweets and chemicals. As a result, our taste buds have become warped as we have come to crave the "highs" of sugar, fat and salt which have become a standard part of the typical American diet. In fact, our taste buds are really driving our cancers.

By following the RAVE Diet, your taste buds will be "re-trained" and the cravings you have for bad foods will be replaced with a desire to eat good food. This is the essence of the RAVE Diet: re-training your taste buds to enjoy the plant foods nature provided for us throughout our history. Once your taste buds are re-oriented, all the health benefits of this diet will fall into place automatically as your body begins to heal.

Many people made a switch from whole milk to skim milk. Do you remember how terrible skim milk tasted when you first tried it? Once you got used to skim milk – and you tried whole milk again – do you remember how awful it tasted? Too heavy, too greasy and too fatty. You will experience similar changes in taste when switching to the RAVE Diet. The highs of sugar, fat, sweets and chemical additives will be replaced by more subtle tastes, along with the aromatic flavors of herbs, spices and sauces. Food will taste much cleaner, much like the difference between spring water and a syrupy soda.

The RAVE Diet is actually pretty simple in terms of re-training your tastes because we're already familiar with most of the foods in the diet. The big difference is that we have to eat *more* of them, then gradually try out unfamiliar foods and discover interesting new tastes.

You'll find you actually have a wide range of food choices "doin' the RAVE," and in the process you'll discover just how narrow your old eating habits actually were. It's an old-fashioned diet, but with some significant improvements. Think of it as an adventure not only in food, but also in health, that will have profound paybacks over the years.

The word RAVE is a simple acronym used to help people remember the rules. It is based on the guidelines used by doctors to treat and reverse diseases. This is what RAVE stands for:

No **R** efined foods
No **A** nimal foods
No **V** egetable oils
No **E** xceptions
   & Exercise

The following sections provide a succinct explanation.

No Refined Foods

"Unhealthy food is available everywhere all the time, like never before in history. Gas stations, drug stores, schools…" – Dr. Kelly D. Brownell, Yale University

"Hunters are using candy as bear bait. After gorging himself on candy, one bear just started walking around in circles…. Among the deleterious health effects: cavities, hair loss and lethargy. If it does that to a 500 pound bear, just imagine what it does to humans." – Newsweek, November 3, 2003

Refined foods are plant foods that have been denatured and stripped of their fiber, vitamins, minerals, antioxidants and other micronutrients. These foods are lifeless imitations of the vibrant products found in nature. They are devoid of any nutritional value and are usually transformed into dull, man-made foodstuffs that do not satisfy hunger, wreak havoc on our health and generally don't require teeth to eat them. Sadly, about *half* of the total calories in a typical American diet come from refined foods.

Refined foods are *simple* carbohydrates such as white flour, wheat flour, refined sugar, pastries, white pasta, white semolina, white bread, white rice (literally any food that's white), French fries, chips of any variety, cakes, soft drinks and similar junk foods. You know the foods I'm talking about – foods that have been transformed from their natural state into man-made products. (See *Reading Labels & Ingredients*.)

This includes refined soy- or rice-based meat and milk substitutes (e.g., soy/rice milk, tofu, etc.). The only soy product allowed on this diet is the whole soy bean (endamame). The only rice product allowed is whole brown rice. (See *Notes - Soy and Breast Cancer* for more on soy.)

Because refined foods have no fiber, they spike your blood sugar, cause insulin surges, stimulate your appetite, accelerate the conversion of calories into body fat and promote many diseases. From your body's perspective, eating refined foods is, for all practical purposes, the same thing as eating refined sugar. Refined foods do not fill you up, so you'll be hungry shortly after eating them, which means you'll have to eat even more empty calories to feel full.

Many people think they are eating a plant-based diet because they are eating foods that do not contain animal products. Refined foods are every bit as bad for your body as animal foods and should be eliminated from your diet. A plant-based diet is about eating natural, whole plant foods. The health benefits of this diet will be greatly diminished if refined foods are not eliminated.

Food manufacturers have spent billions of dollars researching ways to mix the right ingredients in order to "seduce" you into eating bad foods. Scientists have found that chocolate, for example, reaches its point of "maximum irresistibility" with a mix of 50 percent sugar and 50 percent fat.[4] But it doesn't stop there. Ingredient profiles have been created that are targeted at genders and age groups in order to make refined foods as addicting as possible. If this reminds you of cigarette companies, you're thinking in the right direction.

Americans now spend about 90 percent of their food budget on refined foods. As a result of processing foods, the natural flavor is destroyed and has to be replaced with chemical additives. In fact, the heart of food flavor in America does not come from natural foods at all, but from the refineries and chemical plants that dot an industrial corridor along the New Jersey turnpike.

Chemical flavoring not only accounts for the flavor in refined foods, but also in most of the meat Americans consume. Eric Schlosser documents this flavoring via chemistry with the following account:

> "After closing my eyes, I suddenly smelled a grilled hamburger. The aroma was uncanny, almost miraculous. It smelled like someone in the room was flipping burgers on a hot grill. But when I opened my eyes, there was just a narrow strip of white paper [under my nose] and a smiling flavorist."[5]

Ninety percent of the money Americans shell out for food purchases a mix of chemistry and fiber-less, processed foodstuffs devoid of any real nutritional merit. This is how removed we have become from real food (and how we've become so malnourished). We have not only lost our taste for real food, but we've come to prefer the taste of chemicals. If that isn't bad enough, 75 percent of all refined foods – from sodas to soups – contain genetically engineered ingredients, particularly refined soy products.

As opposed to the *simple carbohydrates* found in refined foods, *complex carbohydrates* are found in natural, whole foods, such as whole grains, vegetables and fruits. These are the good carbohydrates that keep your blood sugar level on an even keel, promote health and keep you feeling full longer because they contain their natural fiber and all the nutrients nature gave them.

---

[4] Breaking the Food Seduction, Neal Barnard, M.D., p. 46.
[5] Fast Food Nation, Eric Schlosser, p. 129.

Always use *whole* wheat pastas or *whole* wheat breads because they've kept their fiber on the way to the grocery store. Make sure the label says _whole_ wheat, *not* wheat flour. With grain products, *the first ingredient should always have the word "whole" in it*, sprouted wheat or organic rolled oats. Don't let the words "hearty wheat," "stoned wheat," or "multigrain" on the package fool you. This is just healthy-sounding advertising because these ingredients are made from refined white flour. And there is no difference between white flour and wheat flour. Wheat flour has some caramel coloring so it looks brown and sounds healthier, but it's the same as white flour.

Those who complain about carbohydrates are complaining about *refined*, or simple, carbohydrates, not the *complex carbohydrates* found in whole, natural foods. Those in pursuit of weight loss on "low-carb" diets are trading one set of problems for another because their diets are lacking in nutrients, particularly micronutrients. This is one reason why low-carb diets recommend that people take supplements – in order to try to make up for the poor nutrition of such diets.

Plant fiber does a number of miraculous things for your health, but one thing it does best is remove toxic substances from your body so you can flush them down the toilet. Fiber even removes heavy metals such as mercury, which you probably have in your body as a result of eating fish, or farm animals that were fed fishmeal. Fiber also removes cholesterol – the reason a fiber-rich diet will lower your cholesterol. In addition, fiber binds with sex hormones, such as estrogen, and removes them from your body. In the case of estrogen, American women have very high levels of estrogen due not only to our high-fat diet, but also due to the lack of fiber in our diets. Fiber also slows down glucose absorption. This is very important because surges in glucose will feed cancer cells. Fiber also controls the rate of digestion, making food act more like a time-release pill, which will keep you feeling full.[6]

Think of plant fiber as your intestinal broom because it will clean out a dirty colon and prevent bad things from happening, like cancer. One of the major reasons refined foods and animal foods are not part of the RAVE Diet is because neither of these foods contain fiber.

If you don't think you're eating much refined food now, I have a small experiment for you. All refined foods come in some kind of packaging. Every time you eat any refined food, keep the packaging it came in and put it in a bag. Do this for a week and at the end of the week inspect the contents of the bag. That should be enough to scare you into eliminating refined foods from your diet.

---

[6] These are just a few of the things fiber does for you. It's interesting to note that in 1969, the same year Americans put a man on the moon, our most distinguished nutrition experts thought fiber played no role in human health, that it was just excess baggage plant foods carried around with them.

No Animal Foods

"Cancer is most frequent where carnivorous habits prevail."
– Scientific American, 1892

"When we kill animals to eat them, they end up killing us because their flesh, which contains cholesterol and saturated fat, was never intended for human beings, who are natural herbivores." – William Clifford Roberts, M.D., Editor-in-Chief, American Journal of Cardiology

"No one can contemplate directly eating 13 pats of butter, but they essentially do when they eat a cheeseburger."
– William Connor, M.D., The New American Diet

All animal foods are excluded from the RAVE Diet because they promote cancer. The link between animal foods and cancer begins back in 1892 with a study published in the Scientific American, from which the quote above is taken. Subsequently, there has been a mountain of evidence compiled that confirms this link.[7]

---

[7] A small sampling: Skog KI, Johansson MAE, Jagerstad MI. Carcinogenic heterocyclic amines in model systems and cooked foods: a review on formation, occurrence, and intake. Food and Chem Toxicol 1998;36:879-96; Cummings JH, Bingham SA. Diet and the prevention of cancer. BMJ 1998;317:1636-40; Doll R, Peto R. The causes of cancer: quantitative estimates of avoidable risks of cancer in the United States today. J Natl Canc Inst 1981;66:1191-308; Kromhout D. Essential micronutrients in relation to carcinogenesis. Am J Clin Nutr 1987;45:1361-7; Munoz de Chavez M, Chavez A. Diet that prevents cancer: recommendations from the American Institute for Cancer Research. Int J Cancer Suppl 1998;11:85-9; Makinodan T, Lubinski J, Fong TC. Cellular, biochemical, and molecular basis of T-cell senescence. Arch Pathol Lab Med 1987;111:910-4; Chandra S, Chandra RK. Nutrition, immune response, and outcome. Progress in Food and Nutrition Science 1986;10:1-65; Barone J, Hebert JR, Reddy MM. Dietary fat and natural-killer cell activity. Am J Clin Nutr 1989;50:861-7; Nordenstrom J, Jarstrand C, Wiernik A. Decreased chemotactic and random migration of leukocytes during intralipid infusion. Am J Clin Nutr 1979;32:2416-22; Malter M, Schriever G, Eilber U. Natural killer cells, vitamins, and other brood components of vegetarian and omnivorous men. Nutr Cancer 1 989;12:271-8; Lauffer RB. Iron Balance. New York, NY: St. Martin's Press, 1991; Armstrong B, Doll R. Environmental factors and cancer incidence and mortality in different countries, with special reference to dietary practices. Int J Cancer 1975;15:617-31; Hirayama T. Epidemiology of breast cancer with special reference to the role of diet. Prev Med 1978;7:173-95; Lands WEM, Hamazaki T, Yamazaki K, et al. Changing dietary patterns. Am J Clin Nutr 1990;51:991-3; Carroll KK, Braden LM. Dietary fat and mammary carcinogenesis. Nutrition and Cancer

1985;6:254-9; Rose DP, Boyar AP, Wynder EL. International comparisons of mortality rates for cancer of the breast, ovary, prostate, and colon, and per capita food consumption. Cancer 1986;58:2363-71; U.S. Department of Health and Human Services. Surgeon General's Report on Nutrition and Health. DHHS Publ No. 88-50210, 1988; Rose DP, Boyar AP, Cohen C, Strong LE. Effect of a low-fat diet on hormone levels in women with cystic breast disease. 1. Serum steroids and gonadotropins. J Natl Cancer Inst 1987;78(4):623-6; Ingram DM, Bennett FC, Willcox D, de Klerk N. Effect of low-fat diet on female sex hormone levels. J Natl Cancer Inst 1987;79:1225-9; Goldin BR, Gorbach SL. Effect of diet on the plasma levels, metabolism and excretion of estrogens. Am J Clin Nutr 1988;48:787-90; Toniolo P, Riboli E, Protta F, Charrel M, Cappa AP. Calorie-providing nutrients and risk of breast cancer. J Natl Cancer Inst 1989;81:278; Robbana-Barnat S, Rabache M, Rialland E, Fradin J. Heterocyclic amines: occurrence and prevention in cooked food. Environ Health Perspect 1996;104:280-8; Thiebaud HP, Knize MG, Kuzmicky PA, Hsieh DP, Felton JS. Airborne mutagens produced by frying beef, pork, and a soy-based food. Food Chem Toxicol 1995;33(10):821-8; De Stefani E, Ronco A, Mendilaharsu M, Guidobono M, Deneo-Pellegrini H. Meat intake, heterocyclic amines, and risk of breast cancer: a case-control study in Uruguay. Cancer Epidemiol Biomarkers Prev 1997;6(8):573-81; Matos EL, Thomas DB, Sobel N, Vuoto D. Breast cancer in Argentina: case-control study with special reference to meat eating habits. Neoplasma 1991;38(3):357-66; Howe GR, Hirohata T, Hislop T, et al. Dietary factors and risk of breast cancer: combined analysis of 12 case-control studies. J Natl Cancer Inst 1990;82:561-9; Lubin F, Ruder AM, Wax Y, Modan B. Overweight and changes in weight throughout adult life in breast cancer etiology. Am J Epidemiol 1985;122:579-88; Elwood JM, Cole P, Rothman KJ, Kaplan SD. Epidemiology of endometrial cancer. J Natl Cancer Inst 1977;59:1055-60; Carter BS, Carter HB, Isaacs JT. Epidemiologic evidence regarding predisposing factors to prostate cancer. Prostate 1990;16:187-97; Howell MA. Factor analysis of international cancer mortality data and per capita food consumption. Br J Cancer 1974;29:328-36; Kolonel LN, Hankin JH, Lee J, Chu SY, Nomura AMY, Hinds MW. Nutrient intakes in relation to cancer incidence in Hawaii. Br J Cancer 1981;44:332-9; Rotkin ID. Studies in the epidemiology of prostatic cancer: expanded sampling. Cancer Treat Rep 1977;61:173-80; Schuman LM, Mandel JS, Radke A, Seal U, Halberg F. Some selected features of the epidemiology of prostatic cancer: Minneapolis-St. Paul, Minnesota case control study, 1976-1979. In: Magnus K, ed. Trends in Cancer Incidence: Causes and Practical Implications. Washington, DC: Hemisphere Publishing Corp., 1982; Graham S, Haughey B, Marshall J, et al. Diet in the epidemiology of carcinoma of the prostate gland. J Natl Cancer Inst 1983;70:687-92; Ross RK, Shimizu H, Paganini-Hill A, Honda G, Henderson BE. Case-control studies of prostate cancer in blacks and whites in Southern California. J Natl Cancer Inst 1987;78:869-74; Severson RK, Nomura AM, Grove JS, Stemmermann GN. A prospective study of demographics, diet, and prostate cancer among men of Japanese ancestry in Hawaii. Cancer Research 1989;49:1857-60; Oishi K, Okada K, Yoshida O, et al. A case control study of prostatic cancer with reference to dietary habits. Prostate 1988;12:179-90; Mettlin C, Selenskas S, Natarajan N, Huben R. Beta-carotene and animal fats and their relationship to prostate cancer risk: a case-control study. Cancer 1989;64:605-12; Hirayama T. Epidemiology of prostate cancer with special reference to the role of diet. Natl Cancer Inst Monogr 1979;53:149-54; Phillips RL. Role of lifestyle and dietary habits in risk of cancer among Seventh-day Adventists. Cancer Research

Aside from what's been previously discussed, some of the more interesting evidence concerns the role of animal protein in the promotion of cancer. In the 1960's, researchers in India thought by increasing animal protein, it would actually help cure cancer. What they found was just the opposite. In 100 percent of the cases, increasing the consumption of animal protein *caused* cancer.[8] During the 1980s, Dr. Robert Good, discovered that mice which were fed a low protein diet had fewer cancers. He followed this up by studying the low-protein diets of aborigines in Australia, who had extremely low rates of cancer.[9] Most recently, Dr. T. Colin Campbell[10] has also confirmed the animal protein-cancer connection, but with more precision and depth. Following the lead of the researchers in India, he injected rats with a powerful carcinogen (aflatoxin) to induce liver cancer.[11] When they were fed a 20 percent animal protein diet, *100 percent* of them developed cancer. When they were fed a five percent animal

---

1975;35:3513-22; Mills P, Beeson WL, Phillips RL, Fraser GE. Cohort study of diet, lifestyle, and prostate cancer in Adventist men. Cancer 1989;64:598-604; Willett WC, Stampfer MJ, Colditz GA, Rosner BA, Speizer FE. Relation of meat, fat, and fiber intake to the risk of colon cancer in a prospective study among women. N Engl J Med 1990;323:1664-72; Gerhardsson de Verdier M, Hagman U, Peters RK, Steineck G, Overvik E. Meat, cooking methods, and colorectal cancer: a case-referent study in Stockholm. Int J Cancer 1991;49:520-5; Singh PN, Fraser GE. Dietary risk factors for colon cancer in a low-risk population. Am J Epidemiol 1998;148(8):761-74; Giovannucci E, Rimm EB, Stampfer MJ, Colditz GA, Ascherio A, Willett WC. Intake of fat, meat, and fiber in relation to risk of colon cancer. Cancer Res 1994;54(9):2390-7; World Cancer Research Fund. Food, Nutrition, and the Prevention of Cancer: A Global Perspective. American Institute of Cancer Research. Washington, DC: 1997; Gregorio DI, Emrich LJ, Graham S, Marshall JR, Nemoto T. Dietary fat consumption and survival among women with breast cancer. J Natl Cancer Inst 1985;75:37-41; Verreault R, Brisson J, Deschenes L, Naud F, Meyer F, Belanger L. Dietary fat in relation to prognostic indicators in breast cancer. J Natl Cancer Inst 1988;80:819-25; Newman SC, Miller AB, Howe CR. A study of the effect of weight and dietary fat on breast cancer survival time. Am J Epidemiol 1986;123:767-74; Holm LE, Callmer E, Hjalmar ML, Lidbrink E, Nilsson B, Skoog L. Dietary habits and prognostic factors in breast cancer. J Natl Cancer Inst 1989;81:1218-23; Donegan WL, Hartz AJ, Rimm AA. The association of body weight with recurrent cancer of the breast. Cancer 1978;41:1590-4; Schapira DV, Kumar NB, Lyman GH, Cox CE. Obesity and body fat distribution and breast cancer prognosis. Cancer 1991;67:523-8.

[8] Madhavan TV, and Gopalan C., The effect of dietary protein on carcinogenesis of aflatoxin." Arch. Path. 85 (1968): 133-137.

[9] Good, Robert A., Fernandes, Gabriel, and Day, Noorbibi D., The Influence of Nutrition on Development of Cancer Immunity and Resistance to Mesenchymal Diseases, 1982, New York Raven Press, Molecular Interrelations of Nutrition and Cancer; A New Cancer Link:Gene-Pool Pollution," Modern Medicine, 11/29/71, p. 13; Diet Linked to Cancer Control, San Francisco Chronicle, 10/21/71.

[10] T. Colin Campbell, Ph.D. and Thomas M. Campbell II, The China Study.

[11] Dunaif, GE, Campbell TC, Dietary Protein level and aflatoxin B1-induced preneoplastic hepatic lesions in the rat. Nutrition 117 No. 7, 1987: 1298-302.

protein diet, none of them developed cancer. Dr. Campbell found that cancer could actually be turned on and off by simply changing the amount of animal protein in the diet.

In contrast, when the animals were fed a diet of 20 percent *vegetable* protein, *none of them developed cancer*, despite the presence of the carcinogen. Cancer was only triggered with animal protein, above a threshold of about eight percent of total calories. In further experiments, he found that regardless of how many carcinogens entered the body, the development of cancer was totally dependent on how much animal protein was present, *not the amount of carcinogens*. In other words, the animal protein served to "fertilize" the carcinogens and trigger the onset of cancer. In the absence of animal protein (or at very low levels), cancers were not triggered.

Dr. Campbell did his studies using dairy protein (casein), but he also investigated whether nutrients other than dairy protein might promote or reverse cancers. With stunning consistency, nutrients from *all animal foods grew tumors*, while nutrients from *all plant foods shrank tumors*.

In yet further tests, it was found that casein, the primary protein in all dairy products, was the most aggressive cancer promoter of all.[12]

How well do these laboratory studies translate into human terms? Dr. Campbell has two answers. The first is that although his studies were with rats, the biochemistry of cancer causation between rats and humans is the same.[13] Second, he directed the largest nutritional study ever conducted in human history, The China Project.[14] After detailed analysis of dietary patterns, down to the village level, he concluded that differences in cancer rates corresponded directly to differences in the amount of animal protein consumed: The more animal protein, the more cancer.

Another reason why animal protein causes cancer has to do with digestive enzymes – or a shortage of them as a result of eating animal foods.[15] Cancer cells have a protective protein coating around them which makes them *invisible* to the immune system. The pancreas produces two enzymes[16] that help digest animal protein. In addition to digesting animal protein, only these enzymes can dissolve the protein coating around cancer cells. Once the protein coating is dissolved by the enzymes, the cancer cells become *visible* and the immune system can do its job of destroying them.

---

[12] Inhibition of hepatocellular carcinoma development in hepatitis B virus transfected mice by low dietary casein, Cheng, Z, Hu, J., King, J., et al., Hepatology 26 No. 5 (1997: 1351-54).

[13] From an interview with T. Colin Campbell in the film, Healing Cancer From Inside Out by Mike Anderson.

[14] More information can be found at www.nutrition.cornell.edu/chinaproject/.

[15] This was first documented by Dr. John Beard in his book published in 1911, The Enzyme Treatment of Cancer And Its Scientific Basis. For more information, see the write up in Richard Walters, Options - The Alternative Cancer Therapy Book.

[16] Trypsin and chymotripsin.

Animal protein requires a lot of enzymes to digest it and eating a diet high in animal protein can cause a shortage of pancreatic enzymes. When this happens, cancer cells will keep their protective protein coating and remain invisible to the immune system – and start multiplying throughout the body. The more animal protein you eat, in other words, the more you impair your body's natural defenses against cancer.

In contrast, pancreatic enzymes are not necessary to digest vegetable protein – so you can eat as much vegetable protein as you want and the supply of pancreatic enzymes available to unmask cancer cells will be remain plentiful.

Therapies based on pancreatic enzyme supplementation have been successful in treating cancer,[17] but it's much easier, cheaper and healthier to simply eliminate animal products from your diet.

These findings fit together with Dr. Campbell's findings: Animal protein promotes cancer and vegetable protein does not. In fact, vegetable protein does just the opposite: it fights cancer. These findings also agree with thousands of studies linking animal-based diets with cancer. What's amazing is that it has taken all these studies to confirm what was obvious to observers in the 1890s.

Cancer is very rare in areas of the world where people eat low-fat, plant-based diets. There is 120 times less incidence of prostate cancer, for example, in China compared to the United States.[18] As the Chinese change to the Western diet, however, their risk increases proportionally with their higher intake of animal foods.[19] This was demonstrated in a study in China where they found a man's chance for developing prostate cancer increased directly with the increased consumption of animal products.[20] Migration studies have also shown that as people leave their low-fat, plant-based diets behind and adopt the standard American diet and lifestyle, their risk of cancer increases with each year of residence in their new country.[21]

You do not need animal foods or "complete proteins" and you are much better off in all ways when you avoid them altogether. You will also get more than

---

[17] One of the main practitioners of this type of therapy is Dr. Nicolas Gonzales. For more information see www.dr-gonzalez.com/. For a recent news article on this see www.msnbc.msn.com/id/20164234/.

[18] Wang Y. Decreased growth of established human prostate LNCaP tumors in nude mice fed a low-fat diet. J Natl Cancer Inst. 1995 Oct 4;87(19):1456-62. As noted previously, it is invariably the upper classes in such countries which get cancers because they can afford to eat animal foods.

[19] Sung JF. Risk factors for prostate carcinoma in Taiwan: a case-control study in a Chinese population. Cancer. 1999 Aug 1;86(3):484-91.

[20] Lee MM. Case-control study of diet and prostate cancer in China. Cancer Causes Control. 1998 Dec;9(6):545-52.

[21] For example, see Whittemore AS. Prostate cancer in relation to diet, physical activity, and body size in blacks, whites, and Asians in the United States and Canada. J Natl Cancer Inst. 1995 May 3;87(9):652-61.

enough protein on this diet. If you are concerned about protein issues, see *Part 3 – Protein* for more on this.

You are trying to rebuild your body and eating animal foods not only promotes cancer, but cardiovascular and a host of other diseases. You are trying to get the biochemistry of your body back into balance, but animal foods will unbalance it because they contain high levels of:

- Fat
- Cholesterol
- Protein
- Sodium
- Iron
- Toxins
- Arachidonic acids (turned into prostaglandins, linked to cancer)
- Lead, cadmium, mercury and other metals
- Hormones and antibiotics

Animal foods are also much harder to digest than plant foods, which cause your digestive system to work harder. As a result, there will be less energy available for healing. On top of that, the nitrogenous breakdown products of protein metabolism irritate the immune system and consume its resources.

With respect to some cancers, there is a little known problem with eating meat and dairy: 89 percent of the herds in the U.S. are infected with the leukemia virus, which causes leukemia and lymphomas in cows.[22] This isn't just an American problem as 84% of herds in Argentina and 70% in Canada also have the bovine leukemia virus,[23] as well as high percentages in other meat-eating countries throughout the world. Some countries, such as Finland, have thoroughly eliminated the virus from their cattle, after some 30 years of effort.[24] In the study cited above, regarding American cattle, researchers found that 74 percent of the people they tested had been infected by this bovine virus, due to their meat- and dairy-based diets.

---

[22] Buehring GC, Philpott SM, Choi KY. Humans have antibodies reactive with Bovine leukemia virus. AIDS Res Hum Retroviruses. 2003 Dec;19(12):1105-13.
[23] Sargeant JM. Associations between farm management practices, productivity, and bovine leukemia virus infection in Ontario dairy herds. Prev Vet Med. 1997 Aug;31(3-4):211-21; VanLeeuwen JA,. Seroprevalence of infection with Mycobacterium avium subspecies paratuberculosis, bovine leukemia virus, and bovine viral diarrhea virus in maritime Canada dairy cattle. Can Vet J. 2001 Mar;42(3):193-8; Trono KG. Seroprevalence of bovine leukemia virus in dairy cattle in Argentina: comparison of sensitivity and specificity of different detection methods. Vet Microbiol. 2001 Nov 26;83(3):235-48.
[24] Nuotio L, Rusanen H, Sihvonen L, Neuvonen E. Eradication of enzootic bovine leukosis from Finland. Prev Vet Med. 2003 May 30;59(1-2):43-9.

In addition to infecting white blood cells, these bovine viruses also attack other cells in the body, such as cells of the breast and the lymph nodes. One study found the virus in the breast tissues of 10 of 23 human breast cancer patients.[25]

In America and worldwide, leukemia and lymphoma are much more common in populations consuming higher amounts of dairy and beef,[26] particularly among dairy farmers,[27] while people working in occupations associated with cattle have twice the risk of developing leukemia and lymphoma.[28]

Each year about 30,000 new cases of leukemia and 70,000 new cases of lymphoma occur for "unknown reasons" in the U.S., and undoubtedly many are caused by the bovine virus. The best way to protect yourself against this virus, even if you already have it, is to avoid meat and dairy products and eat the RAVE way, as it's been shown to greatly reduce your risk of being infected.[29]

---

[25] GC Buehring, KY Choi and HM Jensen. Bovine leukemia virus in human breast tissues. Breast Cancer Res 2001, 3(Suppl 1):A14; Buehring GC   Evidence of bovine leukemia virus in human mammary epithelial cells Semin Cell Dev Biol 199735: 27A; Abstract V-1001.

[26] Sarasua S, Savitz DA. Cured and broiled meat consumption in relation to childhood cancer: Denver, Colorado (United States). Cancer Causes Control. 1994 Mar;5(2):141-8; Zhang S, Hunter DJ, Rosner BA, Colditz GA, Fuchs CS, Speizer FE, Willett WC. Dietary fat and protein in relation to risk of non-Hodgkin's lymphoma among women. J Natl Cancer Inst. 1999 Oct 20;91(20):1751-8; Fritschi L, Johnson KC, Kliewer EV, Fry R; Canadian Cancer Registries Epidemiology Research Group. Animal-related occupations and the risk of leukemia, myeloma, and non-Hodgkin's lymphoma in Canada. Cancer Causes Control. 2002 Aug;13(6):563-71; Chiu BC. Diet and risk of non-Hodgkin lymphoma in older women. JAMA. 1996 May 1;275(17):1315-21; Cunningham AS. Lymphomas and animal-protein consumption. Lancet. 1976 Nov 27;2(7996):1184-6.

[27] Hursting SD. Diet and human leukemia: an analysis of international data. Prev Med. 1993 May;22(3):409-22; Howell MA. Factor analysis of international cancer mortality data and per capita food consumption. Br J Cancer. 1974 Apr;29(4):328-36; Kristensen P. Incidence and risk factors of cancer among men and women in Norwegian agriculture. Scand J Work Environ Health. 1996 Feb;22(1):14-26; Reif J. Cancer risks in New Zealand farmers. Int J Epidemiol. 1989 Dec;18(4):768-74; Blair A. Leukemia cell types and agricultural practices in Nebraska. Arch Environ Health. 1985 Jul-Aug;40(4):211-4; Donham KJ. Epidemiologic relationships of the bovine population and human leukemia in Iowa. Am J Epidemiol. 1980 Jul;112(1):80-92.

[28] Fritschi L, Johnson KC, Kliewer EV, Fry R; Canadian Cancer Registries Epidemiology Research Group. Animal-related occupations and the risk of leukemia, myeloma, and non-Hodgkin's lymphoma in Canada. Cancer Causes Control. 2002 Aug;13(6):563-71.

[29] Zhang SM, Hunter DJ, Rosner BA, Giovannucci EL, Colditz GA, Speizer FE, Willett WC. Intakes of fruits, vegetables, and related nutrients and the risk of non-Hodgkin's lymphoma among women. Cancer Epidemiol Biomarkers Prev. 2000 May;9(5):477-85; Marilyn L. Kwan, Gladys Block, Steve Selvin, Stacy Month, and Patricia A. Buffler. Food Consumption by Children and the Risk of Childhood Acute Leukemia. Am. J. Epidemiol. 2004 160: 1098-1107.

As mentioned before, there is a very strong relationship between dairy and hormonal cancers. Prostate cancer, for example, is more strongly related to the consumption of nonfat dairy products than to any other food.[30] In one study, it was shown that high consumption of dairy products was associated with a 50 percent increase in the risk of prostate cancer.[31] One possible reason for this involves vitamin D, which is known to protect against cancer. Consuming high levels of calcium, as found in dairy foods, lowers the levels of vitamin D and in doing so, lowers its cancer-protective qualities.

Another mechanism linking dairy with hormonal cancers is the powerful growth-stimulating hormone known as insulin-like growth factor-1 (IGF-1), which has been strongly linked to the development of cancer of the breast, prostate, lung and colon because it stimulates cell proliferation and inhibits cell death – two activities you don't want when cancer cells are involved.[32] This hormone is increased in the body by the consumption of protein, and especially animal protein. Dairy products stimulate the production of IGF-1 more than any other food.[33]

Some people think they can defeat cancer by eating "organic" animal products. No doubt they are better in a few ways, but saying organic animal products are better for you, is like saying organic tobacco is better for smokers. Animal protein is animal protein, saturated fat is saturated fat, whether it's organic or not. Organic animal foods will plug up your arteries and promote cancer just as fast as non-organic animal foods.

Others may argue that "raw" animal foods are better for you. Nonsense. In fact, T. Colin Campbell did his experiments using raw animal food, which produced cancer reliably and predictably. So, too, did the researchers in India. Animal foods create the same mischief whether they are cooked or not.

The only thing you'll miss from not eating animal foods is the saturated fat, cholesterol and animal proteins – as well as the diseases these ingredients bring to your body. When you come right down to it, all our nutrients are ultimately obtained from plant foods. Meat-eating animals (including humans) feed off plant-eating animals. These animals really amount to storage systems for plant nutrients. The problem, of course, is that the plant nutrients in animals are

---

[30] Grant WB. An ecologic study of dietary links to prostate cancer. Altern Med Rev. 1999 Jun;4(3):162-9

[31] Chan JM. Dairy products, calcium, phosphorous, vitamin D, and risk of prostate cancer (Sweden) Cancer Causes Control. 1998 Dec;9(6):559-66. For the role of meat and IGF, see Andrew W. Roddam, et al. Insulin-like Growth Factors, Their Binding Proteins, and Prostate Cancer Risk. Annals of Internal Medicine. 7 October 2008, Volume 149, Issue 7, 461-471.

[32] Yu H. Role of the insulin-like growth factor family in cancer development and progression. J Natl Cancer Inst. 2000 Sep 20;92(18):1472-89.

[33] Holmes MD. Dietary Correlates of Plasma Insulin-like Growth Factor I and Insulin-like Growth Factor Binding Protein 3 Concentrations. Cancer Epidemiol Biomarkers Prev 2002 Sep;11(9):852-61.

delivered in a package of saturated fat, cholesterol and animal proteins and most of the cancer-fighting micronutrients have been discarded. So why eat animals when you can get everything you need directly from plants – without the bad stuff – and in a low-fat package with healthy fiber and cancer fighting nutrients to boot?

And calorie for calorie, plant foods are far richer in nutrients than animal foods, with green vegetables being the most nutrient-rich foods on the planet.

From a weight-loss perspective, many studies have confirmed that over time, the more people eat meat, the more they gain weight. The more people eat whole plant foods, the more they lose weight. In a recent multi-nation study, it was found that *without exception*, the thinnest people ate a *complex carbohydrate* diet, while the fattest people ate a meat-based diet.[34] Eliminating meat from your diet is essential if you want to achieve your ideal weight and reverse our major diseases.

If you are already too thin, your concern will obviously be just the opposite: how can I gain weight? We have to step back and think about this for a second. Your body is constantly trying to keep in a state of balance, or homeostasis.[35] Your diet will affect this state of balance, as will drugs and anything else you put into your body. A good diet will bring your body back into balance. Everyone has an ideal weight that can be achieved by bringing his or her body into balance. Those who need to lose weight will lose it and those who need to gain weight, will gain it. As your body heals itself, the weight will come back on as your body returns to normalcy.

From your heart's perspective, the difference between "lighter" meats and red meat is insignificant and much like the difference between regular cigarettes and "light" cigarettes. All meats – from red meat to chicken to turkey to fish to liquid meat (dairy products) – cause degenerative diseases because they all contain high levels of cholesterol, saturated fat and animal protein.

---

[34] Stable behaviors associated with adults' 10-year change in body mass index and likelihood of gain at the waist, H.S. Kahn, L.M. Tatham, C. Rodriguez, et al, Am. J. Public Health 87 (5): 747-57 and American Heart Association Annual Conference on Cardiovascular Disease Epidemiology and Prevention, San Francisco, 2004. American Heart Association news conference; participants: Robert H. Eckel, MD, University of Colorado Health Sciences Center; Randal J. Thomas, MD, Mayo Clinic, Rochester, Minn.; Deborah J. Toobert, PhD, Oregon Research Institute, Eugene, Ore.; Kristie J. Lancaster, PhD, RD, New York University, N.Y.; Alison Jane Rigby, PhD, MPH, RD, Stanford University, Palo Alto, Calif.; and Linda Van Horn, PhD, Northwestern University, Chicago.
[35] Tremblay A. Dietary fat and body weight set point. Nutr Rev. 2004 Jul;62 (7 Pt 2):S75-7; Keesey RE, Hirvonen MD. Body weight set-points: determination and adjustment, J Nutr. 1997 Sep 127(9):1875S-1883S.

So what about fish (or shellfish)[36]? No study has ever demonstrated that fish is heart-healthy.[37] The studies that have been done only show it mitigates the risk of sudden cardiac death among those already suffering heart disease – simply because it's a blood thinner and prevents clotting. This has been translated by the press into somehow preventing heart disease, but that is simply not true. The hype in the press regarding fish is about treating a symptom of heart disease (namely a heart attack) – and prolonging the disease – not preventing, arresting or reversing it. In fact, fish-based diets promote heart disease due to the high levels of cholesterol and saturated fat. Given that, it shouldn't be surprising that eating fish also causes a rise in blood cholesterol levels similar to the rise caused by eating beef and pork.[38]

Men with angina were advised to eat two portions of oily fish each week or take three fish oil capsules daily. They were found to have a higher risk of cardiac death compared to men not given this advice.[39] Patients with coronary heart disease received fish oil capsules for some 28 months. It not only failed to lower their cholesterol, but their arteries closed even more during the study! The authors concluded: "Fish oil treatment for 2 years does not promote major favorable changes in the diameter of atherosclerotic coronary arteries."[40] A review of 48 randomized controlled trials involving over 36,000 participants who took fish oils or ate oily fish found no health benefits from these so-called "healthy fats." The conclusion: "Long chain and shorter chain omega 3 fats do not have a clear effect on total mortality, combined cardiovascular events, or cancer."[41] Men who consumed high levels of fish had a 60 percent increased risk

---

[36] Calorie for calorie, shell fish have high cholesterol levels, as well as high levels of saturated fat, and because they do not move around much, their toxic load is much higher than swimming fish. Some people think shell fish are somehow healthier, but they are not.

[37] Cundiff DK, Lanou AJ, Nigg CR. Relation of omega-3 Fatty Acid intake to other dietary factors known to reduce coronary heart disease risk. Am J Cardiol. 2007 May 1;99(9):1230-3. See also, Katan MB. Fish and heart disease: what is the real story? Nutr Rev 1995 Aug;53(8):228-30.

[38] Davidson MH, Hunninghake D, Maki KC, Kwiterovich PO Jr, Kafonek S. Comparison of the effects of lean red meat vs lean white meat on serum lipid levels among free-living persons with hypercholesterolemia: a long-term, randomized clinical trial. Arch Intern Med. 1999 Jun 28;159(12):1331-8.

[39] Burr ML, Ashfield-Watt PA, Dunstan FD, Fehily AM, Breay P, Ashton T, Zotos PC, Haboubi NA, Elwood PC. Lack of benefit of dietary advice to men with angina: results of a controlled trial. Eur J Clin Nutr. 2003 Feb;57(2):193-200.

[40] Sacks FM, Stone PH, Gibson CM, Silverman DI, Rosner B, Pasternak RC. Controlled trial of fish oil for regression of human coronary atherosclerosis. HARP Research Group. J Am Coll Cardiol. 1995 Jun;25(7):1492-8.

[41] Hooper L, Thompson RL, Harrison RA, Summerbell CD, Ness AR, Moore HJ, Worthington HV, Durrington PN, Higgins JP, Risks and benefits of omega 3 fats for mortality, cardiovascular disease, and cancer: systematic review. BMJ. 2006 Apr 1;332(7544):752-60.

of an acute coronary event and a nearly 70 percent increased risk of cardiovascular death, compared with men who consumed low amounts of fish.[42] In another study, men with high levels of mercury in their bodies had more than double the risk of a heart attack, compared to those with low levels.[43]

The contamination in fish is reason enough not to eat them. Fish and shellfish contain toxic chemicals at concentrations as high as 9 million times more than what was found in the polluted water in which they swim. Tests of fish from U.S. rivers have revealed they contained enough estrogen-mimicking chemicals to promote breast cancer growth,[44] not to mention the high levels of mercury, dioxins and PCB's that are found in fish which are highly associated with cancer and other diseases.

A survey of Lake Michigan fish found that 97 percent of the salmon and 91 percent of the lake trout were heavily contaminated with mercury and all of them were contaminated with PCB's.[45] Little wonder that children exposed to PCB's from Lake Michigan fish tend to have low IQ's, poor reading comprehension, difficulty paying attention and memory problems.[46]

An actress who was eating tuna and other seafood four times a week began experiencing severe headaches, cramping in her fingers and feet, and "…a sort of tingling, as if someone was tickling you, all up and down my body and on my legs, and it got more and more pronounced." She was unable to remember her lines, had crying spells, low-grade depression, loss of memory and brain fog.[47] She had, in fact, mercury poisoning from eating fish. Typical symptoms of mercury exposure include fatigue, headache, joint pain and reduced memory and concentration, but can include nervous system damage and even death.

A survey of over 23,000 postmenopausal women showed that fish consumption was positively associated with higher rates of breast cancer.[48] A number of other studies throughout the years have also shown that eating fish increases the risk of cancer, as well as the risk of the spread of cancer to other

---

[42] Jyrki K. Virtanen, et al. Mercury, Fish Oils, and Risk of Acute Coronary Events and Cardiovascular Disease, Coronary Heart Disease, and All-Cause Mortality in Men in Eastern Finland. Arterioscler. Thromb. Vasc. Biol., Jan 2005; 25: 228 - 233.

[43] Guallar E. Mercury, fish oils, and the risk of myocardial infarction. N Engl J Med. 2002 Nov 28;347(22):1747-54.

[44] Bringing Cancer to the Dinner Table: Breast Cancer Cells Grow Under Influence of Fish Flesh, Scientific American (online), April 17, 2007.

[45] EPA, Lake Michigan Mass Balance, 2004.

[46] Scott Fields, "Great lakes: resource at risk," Environmental Health Perspectives Vol. 113, No. 3 (March 2005), pgs. A164-A173. PCBs have also been linked to altering the sex ratio (the ratio of boys to girls born), reducing fertility, and causing abnormal menstrual cycles in women.

[47] Actress Describes Mercury Poisoning Ordeal, ABCNews, 10/21/05. www.abcnews.go.com/Health/story?id=1235251&page=1

[48] Connie Stripp, et al. Fish Intake Is Positively Associated with Breast Cancer Incidence Rate. J. Nutr. 133:3664-3669, November 2003.

parts of the body.[49] In addition to the high fat levels of fish, fish oils also suppress the immune system.[50]

But even if there were "clean" fish available – and there are not – fish would still not be heart or cancer healthy due to the high levels of saturated fat, cholesterol, animal protein and the lack of fiber, complex carbohydrates and other vitamins.

When you look closely into the health claims of fish, they are in fact, very fishy. The original source of Omega-3 fats is plants and only plants can make Omega-3 fats. Why not get these fats from an uncontaminated source that is good for your health and perfectly balanced in terms of nutrients?

The one sure way we know that animal foods harm us is that our bodies start clearing out our arteries the minute we stop eating them. Dr. Nathan Pritikin, who pioneered heart disease reversal with diet, did not experience success in reversing his heart disease until he completely eliminated animal products from his diet.[51]

Two of the major nutritional weapons in your personal war against cancer are antioxidants and phytochemicals. Where do these come from? Exclusively plant foods. Animal foods are oxidizing agents and have no phytochemicals, except incidentally, because herbivorous animals eat plant foods. I have read articles and books which purport to have anti-cancer diets, yet they recommend eating cancer-promoting animal foods! Any diet which recommends eating animal foods to fight cancer is recommending a "sub-optimal" diet, to be kind, and a just plain dangerous diet, to be unkind.

No Vegetable Oils

Strictly speaking, vegetable oils are part of the Refined Foods group because they contain no fiber, they're devoid of nutrients and they are 100 percent fat. Although I say vegetable oils, because these are what most people consume, I mean *any oils* (e.g., nut oils, coconut oil, etc.).

---

[49] Griffini P. Dietary omega-3 polyunsaturated fatty acids promote colon carcinoma metastasis in rat liver. Cancer Res. 1998 Aug 1;58(15):3312-9; Klieveri L. Promotion of colon cancer metastases in rat liver by fish oil diet is not due to reduced stroma formation. Clin Exp Metastasis. 2000;18(5):371-7; Young MR. Effects of fish oil and corn oil diets on prostaglandin-dependent and myelopoiesis-associated immune suppressor mechanisms of mice bearing metastatic Lewis lung carcinoma tumors. Cancer Res. 1989 Apr 15;49(8):1931-6; Coulombe J. Influence of lipid diets on the number of metastases and ganglioside content of H59 variant tumors. Clin Exp Metastasis. 1997. Jul;15(4):410-7.

[50] Calder PC. Polyunsaturated fatty acids, inflammation, and immunity. Lipids. 2001;36:1007-24.

[51] The Pritikin Program for Diet & Exercise, Nathan Pritikin, M.D., p. 93. See also, the film *Eating* by Mike Anderson for other accounts.

Vegetable oils constitute a whopping 11 percent of the calories Americans consume.[52] Putting two tablespoons of oil in your salad has the fat equivalent of two scoops of ice cream. From a weight loss perspective, eliminating vegetable oils is a very easy – and healthy – way to cut calories. (See *Part 4 – Cooking Without Oil.*)

There are other problems with vegetable oils, however. These oils contain high levels of saturated fat, which is essentially "cholesterol in disguise" because it stimulates your liver to make more cholesterol than your body needs and ends up clogging arteries. In fact, adding *any* oil to your food will raise your cholesterol level even more than eating cholesterol itself.[53]

Hydrogenated vegetable oils (trans-fats) are particularly efficient at clogging arteries and depriving your body of oxygen. These oils are found in all kinds of refined foods such as chips, cookies, crackers, cereals, breakfast bars and other baked goods. Every time you eat a bag of cookies it's no different than biting into a piece of meat, from your body's perspective.

In packaged goods, look for the word "hydrogenated" in the ingredients list and put it back on the shelf. And any food that's deep-fried, such as fast food French fries or donuts, will contain these artery-clogging oils. Many commercial brands of peanut butter also use hydrogenated oils. If you like nut butters, grind your own at a health food store.

Hydrogenated oils are the "glue" that holds refined carbohydrates together in order to increase shelf life. In fact, the healthy amount of trans-fats in your diet should be exactly zero. Ingredients used for longer shelf lives in food translate into longer illnesses and a shorter shelf life for you.

Fried animal foods, such as fried chicken, are probably the *most dangerous foods in existence* because they combine high levels of saturated fat and cholesterol, with high levels of oil. In other words, your blood vessels are getting a triple-whammy when you eat fried animal foods.

Even seemingly "innocent" foods such as movie popcorn are dangerous as they are usually popped in coconut or palm oil, both of which are extremely high in saturated fat.

The current rage among some health authorities is olive oil. It's ironic that our health authorities are advising an overweight nation to eat the most concentrated form of fat on the planet, which packs more calories, pound-for-pound, than butter. The basic reason (presumably) is that they are trying to move people away from margarine, although these same authorities (e.g., The American Heart Association and virtually all major health experts) were praising margarine just a few decades ago – and quoting studies purporting to show margarine, containing hydrogenated oils, was heart-healthy!

---

[52] Eat To Live, Joel Fuhrman, M.D., p. 91.
[53] Dr. Dean Ornish's Program for Reversing Heart Disease, Dean Ornish, M.D., p. 256-257.

Although olive oil is healthier than butter or margarine, that's not saying much. It's probably the worst way to get heart-healthy fats because there's almost no nutritional bang for the calorie buck. In fact, olive and other oils are so nutritionally bankrupt that Joel Fuhrman, M.D., gives oils a score of 1 out of 100, just above refined sweets, which score a zero.[54]

Olive oil is 100 percent fat, contains high concentrations of saturated fat while the fiber, antioxidants, vitamins and minerals of the olive itself have been stripped away. In clinical studies on humans, olive oil has been shown to be as bad for the heart as eating roast beef.[55] In other studies, it has been found that monounsaturated fat, although showing higher HDL and lower LDL levels, resulted in just as much coronary disease as saturated fat.[56]

Using the brachial artery tourniquet test, it was found that olive oil constricted blood flow by a whopping 31 percent![57] Why is this important? Because when arteries constrict, the endothelium (artery's lining) is injured, triggering plaque build-up or arthrosclerosis (heart disease).[58]

In addition, the Omega-3's in vegetable oils are highly unstable and tend to decompose and unleash free radicals that cause damage to cells. Vegetable oils have also been implicated in several different studies with cancers and polyunsaturated fat turn out to be the strongest promoter of skin cancers of all the foodstuffs we eat.[59] Vegetable oils also suppress the immune system and actually promote the spread of some cancers.[60]

---

[54] Eat To Live, Joel Fuhrman, M.D., p. 121.

[55] The Influence of Diet on the Appearance of New Lesions in Human Coronary Arteries, JAMA, 1990, Vol. 263, pp. 1646-52.

[56] Lawrence L. Rudel, et al., Arteriosclerosis, Thrombosis, and Vascular Biology, December, 1995; R. Vogel, et al., Journal of the American College of Cardiology, 2000: The Postprandial Effect of Components of the Mediterranean Diet on Endothelial Function.

[57] Vogel RA. Corretti MC. Plotnick GD. The postprandial effect of components of the Mediterranean diet on endothelial function. Journal of the American College of Cardiology. 36(5):1455-60, 2000 Nov 1.

[58] High fat meals block the endothelium's ability to produce nitric oxide, which is a vasodilator and critical to preserving the tone and health of blood vessels. Moreover, fat should be released into the blood stream slowly and you can only get that slow release by eating natural plant foods in their natural packages that still contain their fiber.

[59] Harris RB, Foote JA, Hakim IA, Bronson DL, Alberts DS. Fatty acid composition of red blood cell membranes and risk of squamous cell carcinoma of the skin. Cancer Epidemiol Biomarkers Prev. 2005 Apr;14(4):906-12. See also John A. McDougall, M.D., www.drmcdougall.com/vegetable_fat.html.

[60] Young MR. Effects of fish oil and corn oil diets on prostaglandin-dependent and myelopoiesis-associated immune suppressor mechanisms of mice bearing metastatic Lewis lung carcinoma tumors. Cancer Res. 1989 Apr 15;49(8):1931-6; Coulombe J. Influence of lipid diets on the number of metastases and ganglioside content of H59 variant tumors. Clin Exp Metastasis. 1997 Jul;15(4):410-7.

Simply put, olive and other vegetable oils are bankrupt foods that have little nutritional value, a very high caloric cost and actually do damage to your body. If you're after the good fat in olives, get it from the olives themselves, not the denatured oil.

Some highly questionable "Mediterranean" diet studies[61] claim to show a "slower progression" of heart disease when people consume olive oil. But having a slower progression of heart disease hardly makes the case that olive oil is heart-healthy, assuming such a causal relationship exists in the first place. Other studies have shown it is not the olive oil at all, but the high fiber content in a traditional Mediterranean-type diet that accounts for lower rates of heart disease.[62] A diet is not heart-healthy unless it arrests and reverses heart disease and only a whole, plant-based diet – which specifically excludes *all* oils – has been proven to do that. Adding oils to such a diet only impairs its effectiveness.

The model for the Mediterranean diet harks back to the 1950s and before when people, especially in the island of Crete, were virtually free of heart disease – despite their indulgence in olive oil. This was not because of the olive oil, but because they ate primarily vegetables and whole grains, a little fish and got lots of exercise. Today, their consumption of olive oil has remained the same (if not increased), but their consumption of whole plant foods has plummeted, as has their exercise. As a result, heart disease and obesity have skyrocketed.[63] Olive oil has nothing to do with preventing heart disease and clinical studies have shown that it promotes arterial lesions.[64] It's just another magic bullet that is a big, fat fantasy promoted by the olive oil industry determined to get high levels of fat back into our diets.

When T. Colin Campbell, author of *The China Study*, was asked what the difference was between the Mediterranean diet and diets in rural China, where heart disease is practically nonexistent, he replied, "I would say the absence of oil in the rural Chinese diet is the reason for their superior success."[65]

---

[61] For example, the Lyon Diet Heart Study. Note that after nearly four years into the study, 25 percent of the subjects following the "heart-healthy" Mediterranean diet had either died or experienced some new cardiovascular event.

[62] European Journal of Clinical Nutrition 2002;56:715-722.

[63] The same sort of argument is made by those peddling any oil. Coconut oil vendors, for example, will argue that despite its very high saturated fat content, populations consuming large quantities of coconut products (such as in the Philippines), have low rates of heart disease. Again, this is due to their overall (traditional) low fat, low cholesterol diet. The low rates of heart disease were achieved not because of the coconut oil, but despite it.

[64] The Influence of Diet on the Appearance of New Lesions in Human Coronary Arteries, JAMA, 1990, Vol. 263, pp. 1646-52.

[65] During a panel discussion at the 2nd National Summit on Cholesterol and Coronary Artery Disease, as quoted in Prevent and Reverse Heart Disease, Caldwell B. Esselstyn, M.D., p. 84.

The leading health authorities in reversing heart disease with diet, including Dr. Caldwell Esselstyn, Dr. Joel Fuhrman, Dr. John McDougall and Dr. Dean Ornish, all agree that vegetable oils should be *excluded* from a heart-healthy diet. These are doctors who actually reverse heart disease, as opposed to those who just talk about it or promote the greasy stuff because of financial ties to the olive oil industry. In fact, there has not been a single case of heart disease arrest or reversal where any vegetable oil was a part of the diet. So, if olive oil is so "heart-healthy," why would doctors who reverse heart disease with diet specifically exclude it? Because they consider vegetable oils to be "heart dangerous" and so should you.

In a nutshell, here's the argument against oils: *All* dietary fats – be they animal or plant fats of all kinds – at levels above 20 percent of total calories, cause heart disease. This has been demonstrated in many clinical tests.[66] In order to prevent heart disease, you have to reduce your *overall* fat intake. A diet of 100 percent whole plant foods is as heart-healthy as you can get. Why introduce a highly concentrated form of fat, such as vegetable oil, that will surely bring your fat intake level into an unsafe zone?

Oils should be put in vehicles and machinery, not your body. In fact, the original use of Canola oil was to lubricate machinery. Then someone came up with the bright idea that people might actually eat it (proving, once again, that people will eat just about anything!). Flaxseed oil is commonly used as a thinner

---

[66] The Influence of Diet on the Appearance of New Lesions in Human Coronary Arteries," D. H. Blankenhorn; R. L. Johnson; W. J. Mack; H. A. el Zein; L. I. Vailas, JAMA, 1990, Vol. 263, pp. 1646-52; Lancet 344:1195, 1994); Aterioscler Thromb Vasc Biol 15:2101, 1995; Dietary Monounsaturated Fatty Acids Promote Aortic Atherosclerosis in LDL Receptor–Null, Human ApoB100–Overexpressing Transgenic Mice, Lawrence L. Rudel, Kathryn Kelley, Janet K. Sawyer, Ramesh Shah, Martha D. Wilson, Arterioscler Thromb Vasc Biol. 1998;18:1818-1827; Combined Intense Lifestyle and Pharmacologic Lipid Treatment Further Reduce Coronary Events and Myocardial Perfusion Abnormalities Compared With Usual-Care Cholesterol-Lowering Drugs in Coronary Artery Disease, Stefano Sdringola, MD, FACC, Keiichi Nakagawa, MD, Yuko Nakagawa, MD, S. Wamique Yusuf, MBBS, MRCP, Fernando Boccalandro, MD, Nizar Mullani, BS, Mary Haynie, RN, MBA, Mary Jane Hess, RN, K. Lance Gould, MD, FACC, Journal of the American College of Cardiology, JACC Vol. 41, No. 2, 2003, 263–72; Effect of Diet on Vascular Reactivity: An Emerging Marker for Vascular Risk, Sheila G. West, Current Atherosclerosis Reports, Vol 3.6, pp. 446-455; Effect of a High-Fat Ketogenic Diet on Plasma Levels of Lipids, Lipoproteins, and Apolipoproteins in Children, Peter O. Kwiterovich, Jr; Eileen P. G. Vining; Paula Pyzik; Richard Skolasky, Jr; John M. Freeman, JAMA. 2003;290:912-920; Rudel LL, Parks JS, Sawyer JK. Compared with dietary monounsaturated and saturated fat, polyunsaturated fat protects African Green Monkeys from coronary artery atherosclerosis. Arterioscler Thromb Vasc Biol 1995;15:2101- 2110; de Lorgeril M, Salen P, Martin JL, Monjaud I, Deloye J, Mamelle N. Mediterranean diet, traditional risk factors, and the rate of cardiovascular complications after myocardial infarction. Circulation 1999;99:779-785.

in paints and varnishes and when consumed in high quantities, can hamper the blood's ability to clot.

Instead of using vegetable oils for cooking, cook at lower temperatures and use water to make your own broth – or use the substitutes below. You'll be surprised at how well they work. And with a little practice, you'll soon find you prefer the cleaner taste. It's like the difference between eating peaches in heavy syrup and eating fresh peaches right off the tree. Once you stop using oils, you will be able to taste the difference and you'll never go back.

Oil substitutes for sautéing: apple juice, sherry, vegetable stock, vinegars, wine, beer.

Oil substitutes in baked goods: applesauce, pureed bananas, pureed stewed prunes.

For salads, choose a dressing without oil or a vinegar-based dressing, such as a Balsamic or brown-rice-seasoned vinegar dressing. Or try citrus juices in place of salad dressing. If you don't like the taste of vinegar dressings, try mixing them with a tomato-based sauce to make your dressing. (See *Part 5 – Salad Dressings Without Oil*.) Many people have started off with this diet and could not stand the taste of vinegar – but now prefer it as because their tastes have changed. Your tastes will change if you give this a chance.

No Exceptions

"We all agree your theory is crazy, but is it crazy enough?"
– Niels Bohr, Nobel Laureate

Now, after all these negative "No's", you're probably thinking I'm crazy for also saying "No Exceptions" because everyone is going to have some exceptions in our world of plentiful temptations. That, however, is precisely why I say it. It's right out of the school of 'if you give them an inch, they'll take a mile.'

Since this book is about providing nutritional support to rebuild your body in order to fight cancer, the No Exceptions rule must be applied to the letter. Success will correspond directly with how strictly you follow the diet.

Doctors who administer dietary treatments to cure diseases will tell you the No Exception rule is the biggest area of concern. When patients stray from their diets, even a little, it can significantly undermine the goals they are trying to achieve.

I can always tell when someone is not following the diet strictly. They will say, "The diet isn't working!" I always volunteer to inspect what's in their refrigerators and pantries – and they *always* say NO! That's because their kitchens are full of exceptions – and so, too, is their diet.

Most of us think we can get away with more than just an occasional exception, but there is real pain involved. "Oh, these are only calories," you say. Ah, but they're not. They're usually *empty* calories, which means you'll soon be hungry again and you'll need to consume even more calories in order to feel full. In addition, it will be a setback to your healing process because your body will have to handle the ingredients you're bringing with the bad food.

Exercise

"The sovereign invigorator of the body is exercise, and of all exercises, walking is the best." – Thomas Jefferson

"It always amazes me that we don't have half an hour to exercise, but manage to squeeze in an average of four hours of TV a day."

"'What, are they allergic to sweat?" – Richard Simmons, fitness personality

Animals in the wild never get fat. Humans in the wild never get fat. Domesticate dogs, they get fat and diseased. Domesticate humans, they get fat and diseased. Our sedentary lifestyles are simply not suited to our Stone Age bodies.

Exercise is an essential part of the RAVE Diet. As mentioned previously, the root of the word diet actually means "lifestyle" and a change in diet really means a change in the style of your life. Active Americans get a fraction of the cancers and other diseases that sedentary Americans get. Among other things, exercise helps to correct bad health habits by burning up and stabilizing blood sugar levels, improving immune function and lymph flow, getting oxygen to all parts of the body and strengthening bones, while helping us handle stress better and increasing both the quality and quantity of sleep.

Exercise also speeds the passage of carcinogens and toxins from the body and recent studies have shown that exercise keeps your brain as fit as your body as you age. In other words, exercise will not only make you feel fit and improve your appearance, but it will prevent a wide range of diseases.

We are aerobic creatures by design. As your main exercise, you should choose a regimen that's just the opposite of cancer – one that's aerobic – an exercise that makes you breathe and respire to raise the oxygen levels in your blood and get your lymphatic system (the body's sewer) flowing to remove waste. It's not a coincidence that lymphatic cancer is one of the fastest growing cancers in the world today due to our increasingly sedentary lifestyle.

Cancer hates oxygen and exercise oxygenates tissues, which slows the progress of anaerobic cancer cells. It also stabilizes blood sugar levels, which selectively deprives cancer cells of their favorite fuel.

Exercise correlates directly with cancer prevention. Of some 959 women with breast cancer, 110 died if they exercised less than three hours a week. In contrast, only 20 died of breast cancer if they exercised three to five hours a week![67]

Early stage breast cancer patients who ate five servings or more a day of vegetables and fruits and walked 30 minutes a day, six days a week, cut their risk of death in half.[68]

Men over the age of 65 who engaged in at least three hours of vigorous physical activity – such as running, biking or swimming – per week had a nearly 70 percent lower risk of being diagnosed with advanced prostate cancer or dying from the disease.[69]

Walking is probably the best exercise for all of us. It's easy, cheap and gets you outdoors, which can do wonders for your mental state. It wasn't that long ago that walking wasn't an exercise at all, but transportation for the vast majority of Americans. Try to find opportunities during the day that allow you to walk more, instead of driving to a destination.

Always get at least half an hour of exercise a day, or 45 minutes five times a week. If you've had a busy day, even 15 minutes can be beneficial. Try walking for 30 minutes in the morning and 30 minutes in the evening. I guarantee it will transform your life within a month.

Get out in the sun occasionally. It will bring some perspective into your life, it's the best way to get vitamin D, and recent studies have shown that moderate exposure has a protective effect against all sorts of cancers – including skin cancer. Just the opposite of what we've been told for the last 20 years. (See *Supplementation – Vitamin D*.)

And when the brain is producing "happy chemicals" – such those released when you exercise – they will actually strengthen your immune system.

The best time to exercise is whenever you can, but most people prefer to exercise in the mornings because it seems to jump-start their metabolism, giving them more energy and mental acuity throughout the day. It's also easier to find the time in the early hours because there are usually fewer demands on your schedule.

Insofar as weight loss is concerned, exercise will reduce fat and build lean muscle mass, which will *increase your metabolism* and that, in turn, will burn more calories. The more exercise you get, the more muscle you gain. The more

---

[67] Michelle D. Holmes, MD, et al. Physical Activity and Survival After Breast Cancer Diagnosis. JAMA, 2005;293:2479-2486. See also, Dorn, J., et al., Lifetime Physical Activity and Breast Cancer Risk in Pre- and Postmenopausal Women. Med. Sci. Sports Exerc., Vol. 35, No. 2, pp. 278-285, 2003.

[68] John P. Pierce, et al. Greater Survival After Breast Cancer in Physically Active Women With High Vegetable-Fruit Intake Regardless of Obesity, JCO Jun 10 2007: 2345-2351.

[69] Giovannucci, E. Archives of Internal Medicine, May 9, 2005: vol 165; pp 1005-1010.

muscle you gain, the more your metabolism and energy will increase – and the more fat you'll burn.

When you're sedentary, you lose muscle mass. When active, you gain it and that is the key to burning more calories. Don't use the excuse that your metabolism slows down with age. Nonsense. Metabolism is a function of lean body mass, the more you have the higher your metabolism. Get moving, build up your lean body mass and your metabolism will move with you.

There's a secret known to those who exercise regularly: Exercise *creates* energy. Don't wait for energy to come to you when you're tired. When you feel that afternoon slump, shake it off and get your body moving. Taking a 15-minute walk will keep you more awake and alert the rest of the day than an afternoon nap – or that cup of coffee.

Humans are naturally lazy because we're programmed to conserve energy. In the past, we were forced to exercise to find food and there was a balance between the calories expended to locate or farm food and the calories we consumed. Today, we have created an incredibly artificial living environment that's also designed to conserve energy. The result is that many Americans are practically living their lives in bed rest! Humans in industrialized countries are very much like caged birds, but in our case we're caged in our chairs and couches. Despite our technical advances, we're still trapped in Stone Age bodies and those bodies need to move – just as faithfully as they are fed every day.

The best incentive to exercise is that it simply makes you feel wonderful and alive! But if you need an immediate reason to exercise, here's one you can't resist – you'll enjoy a much better sex life – and believe it or not, frequent sex is a cancer-fighter![70]

---

[70] Michael F. Leitzmann; Elizabeth A. Platz; Meir J. Stampfer; Walter C. Willett; Edward Giovannucci. Ejaculation Frequency and Subsequent Risk of Prostate Cancer. JAMA. 2004;291:1578-1586.

Essential Dietary Guidelines

Here are a few simple keys to the RAVE Diet.

The #1 Golden Rule: Always eat foods as close to their natural states as possible. Eat whole foods that come in their natural packages and avoid foods that come in a package or can, unless they are fresh-frozen. Some of the sample menus will contain items that are canned. This is for convenience. If you can find the item in its natural state or are willing to take the time to prepare it, then you should do so.

Always eat whole foods: In packaged goods, look for the words "whole," "sprouted wheat" or "organic rolled oats" in the <u>first ingredient</u>, not the second or third. Always eat whole-wheat pastas or whole wheat breads. Make sure the label says whole wheat, <u>not wheat flour</u>. Don't let the words "hearty wheat," "stoned wheat," or "multigrain" on the package fool you. Such ingredients are made from refined white flour and there's no difference between *white* flour and *wheat* flour. Wheat flour has some caramel coloring and sounds healthier, but it's not.

Eat a wide variety of colorful foods: Always eat a wide variety of foods because each food has its own special health benefits and cancer-fighting profiles – and they work as a team, complimenting, reinforcing and magnifying each other's benefits. This is the new math of cancer prevention and eating a variety of foods actually multiplies cancer-fighting and cardiovascular benefits because they work together synergistically. Along the same lines, most of the antioxidant benefits of vegetables come from the component that gives them their color, so make sure your plate is full of different colors – *the deeper and darker the colors, the more cancer-fighting nutrients*. Red leaf lettuce, for example, is much better than pale iceberg lettuce. The magic is in variety. Get in the habit of chopping up vegetables and putting them in containers. That way, you can add a variety of foods to your meal very conveniently.

Greens Should Be an Integral Part of Every Meal: A salad a day keeps the oncologist away – and greens should be part of every meal. In fact, you should never throw away greens, such as the green tops that come with carrots and radishes, because they are far more nutritious – calorie for calorie – than the carrots or radishes themselves. Wash them off and store them in the refrigerator, then add them to juices, smoothies or mix them into other recipes.

Eat Organic Foods: Always eat organic foods. Studies have shown that plant foods contain up to 40 percent – and on average 25 percent – more micronutrients than conventional plant foods grown with chemical fertilizers and pesticides.[71] Getting a higher intake of phytochemicals and antioxidants is the key to battling cancer. Think of micronutrients as millions of "scrubbing bubbles" cleaning up your body, just as the scrubbing bubbles in those commercials cleaned up the bathroom. In addition, organic produce is free of pesticides and genetically modified organisms.

Eat Uncooked Food: *Eat at least half of your food uncooked* and without any dips or toppings, just plain or with herbs and spices. The more uncooked food, the better. In general, cooked or processed foods contain fewer phytochemicals and antioxidants than fresh and uncooked foods.[72] Some nutrients become bioavailable only when you cook food, while others are only available in the food's uncooked state. (For more on this, see *Notes – Raw and Cooked Foods*.) Broccoli and other cruciferous vegetables such as cabbage, kale, Brussels sprouts, radishes and cauliflower are the best sources of a powerful anti-cancer nutrient called sulforaphane. In human tests, the absorption rate of this compound was ten times higher in uncooked broccoli versus cooked broccoli.[73] Steaming is the best way to cook vegetables. Try to eat your food plain. If you buy good-tasting products in the first place, you won't need anything on them. Also include lots of sprouted grains as a regular part of your meals.

A Salad Is An Ideal Meal: A salad puts into practice all of the previous guidelines about eating. Load up on greens. Be careful when eating at a local salad bar, be it in a restaurant or supermarket, because it's unlikely they use organic products. And bring your own salad dressing, or use vinegar without the oil.

No Alcohol: One obvious, but largely ignored refined food is alcohol. Sorry, but you're going on the wagon. For cancer patients, drinking alcohol is particularly dangerous not only because of the high-sugar content, which feeds cancer cells, but because it fuels the production of a growth factor that helps create new blood vessels inside tumors (angiogenesis), which will carry more fuel (glucose) to tumor cells.[74]

---

[71] New Evidence Confirms the Nutritional Superiority of Plant-Based Organic Foods, by Charles Benbrook, Xin Zhao, Jaime Yáñez, Neal Davies and Preston Andrews, March 2008. See www.organic-center.org/reportfiles/5367_Nutrient_Content_SSR_FINAL_V2.pdf.

[72] Henry C, Heppell N (2002). "Nutritional losses and gains during processing: future problems and issues". Proc Nutr Soc 61 (1): 145–8.

[73] Suzanne Dixon, MPH, MS, RD. J Agric Food Chem 2008;56:10505-9.

[74] Jian-Wei Gu, et al., Ethanol stimulates tumor progression and expression of vascular endothelial growth factor in chick embryos, Cancer, Vol. 103, No. 2, 422-431. Researchers injected alcohol into chick embryos and the chicks had eight times more cancer cells in their blood vessels than chicks injected with saline. The researchers also

Chew your food thoroughly: The idea behind nutritional strategies is to give your body a concentrated boost of nutrients. Key to this is the ability to fully digest the foods you are eating, so you get the most nutrients from them. This is where enzymes come into play because enzymes help your body fully digest food. The first step you can take to increase enzyme activity is to chew food very thoroughly because the saliva in your mouth contains enzymes that will break down food and make it more digestible. A good rule of thumb is that your food should be close to liquid before you swallow it, i.e., you should "drink your food." The next place you can get enzymes is by eating uncooked foods. When food is cooked, digestive enzymes are destroyed and so, too, is the ability to get the most nutrients from foods. Eating raw, uncooked food retains the natural enzymes in foods and, thus, your ability to fully absorb their nutrients. This is one reason we say to eat at least half of your food uncooked (above).

Never cook with salt: Natural plant foods contain all the salt you'll ever need. People like to say that salt brings out the flavor in food. Nonsense! All it does is give food a salty taste, camouflage the real taste of food while promoting blood clotting, high blood pressure and a more acidic body. Learn to use spices and herbs, instead of salt, to flavor your food. Or try Mrs. Dash or Salt-Free Spike. A few weeks after you stop using salt, you'll find you won't miss it at all.

Take a Multivitamin or B-12 Supplement: Some people think that having to take a supplement on what is supposedly an "all-natural" diet means it is deficient in some respect, but the opposite is actually the truth. B-12 is a vitamin that is synthesized by bacteria that live in the soil. It does not come from animals. Herbivorous animals happen to have B-12 because they consume soil when they eat plants, thereby storing B-12 in their flesh. Getting enough B-12 was never a problem for our ancestors because they came into contact with the soil constantly. It is only because our environment is so sanitary and our contact with the earth so infrequent that we require this supplement.[75] The recommended daily allowance for B-12 varies by authority, but in general 10 micrograms is more than enough. You will find supplements with 1,000 micrograms or more. This is not a problem because high doses of this vitamin are not toxic.

---

noted significant increases in tumor size and tumor blood vessel density, as well as higher levels of the vascular endothelial growth factor, a protein involved in the growth of new blood vessels (that could feed tumors) in the alcohol-exposed embryos. Although these were large doses of alcohol, the researchers said that based on previous studies, that even light to moderate amounts of alcohol could induce new blood vessel growth for a tumor.
[75] In a few cases, B-12 deficiency has nothing to do with diet because some people who have various stomach disorders cannot make "intrinsic factor," which combines with B-12 and allows it to be absorbed. Certain medicines used to treat stomach acidity can also interfere with B-12 absorption.

Get Adequate Amounts of Vitamin D: If there is a single micronutrient that practically all Americans are deficient in, it is vitamin D, known as the "sunshine" vitamin. The best way to get this vitamin is through exposure to the sun. If you are not able to do this on a regular basis, take a daily vitamin D supplement of 1,000 IU. For details on this, see *Part 3 - Vitamin D*.

Ground Flaxseed: A teaspoon of ground flaxseed should be a part of your daily diet. Flaxseed is not only the single best source of fiber on the planet, but it has been proven to be very effective in fighting breast cancer. It has also been shown to slow the growth of prostate tumors in men[76] and breast tumors in women.[77] Ground flaxseed is cheap and available at health food stores. Keep it in the freezer to prevent the essential fatty acids (Omega-3's) from becoming rancid. Sprinkle it over anything and everything, from salads and oatmeal or any other dish. It is especially good with smoothies and we've made it a part of every smoothie recipe in this book. Avoid flaxseed oil, as it's a refined product and part of the restricted vegetable oil group.

Snacking: Snacking in-between meals is not bad in and of itself; it all depends on what you eat. Avoid packaged "snack" foods like the plague. Always eat whole plant foods when you snack. If you are at work, bring an extra large helping of lunch and snack on that. (See *Part 4 – Fast Food: Meals In Minutes* for quick meal suggestions and *Part 3 – What To Expect* for more on snacking.)

Beverages: Pure water should *always* be your beverage of choice. Any beverage containing any kind of sweetener is off limits. (See *Part 4 – Reading Labels & Ingredients*.) Any beverage containing a stimulant, such as caffeine, is off-limits, as well. Stimulants give you an "artificial" high because when you come down from them, you're at a lower point than you would have been without having taken them in the first place – the reason you need that second cup of coffee. Any stimulant will dehydrate your body and take more fluid out of it than it brings in. This contributes to cell dehydration, which some experts cite as the cause of premature aging.

Blending and juicing is fine, so long as you follow the rules. (See *Part 3 – Green Juicing and Blending*.) There are no specific rules about fluid intake, except that you should drink as much water as you're comfortable with. Avoid "sport drinks" and any drink that carries a "health" label with it. You're simply wasting your money. Of the beverages out there, decaffeinated green tea is

---

[76] Flaxseed, ginseng show benefit in cancer treatment, Reuters, June 4, 2007.
[77] Biological Effects of Dietary Flaxseed In Patients With Breast Cancer, Thompson LU, Li T, Chen J, Goss PE Nutritional Sciences, University of Toronto, Toronto, ON, Canada; Medical Oncology, Princess Margaret Hospital, Toronto, ON, Canada, San Antonio Breast Cancer Symposium 2000.

probably your best bet as it has been amply demonstrated to have anti-cancer and overall health benefits.

Eating Out: Eating out is simply dangerous because you have lost control of the food you put into your mouth. In other words, try to avoid eating out as much as you can. Of course, you can't always do that, so here are some guidelines. Ethnic restaurants usually have the best food choices, but in any restaurant, just order whatever is on the menu, but ask them to leave out the bad stuff by following the RAVE Diet rules. Simply say you don't eat meat and dairy and ask them to prepare a vegetable plate for you. You can request they not cook it in oil, but I've never come across a restaurant chef who knows how to do that. Steamed vegetables are the best. Look at what they are offering as side dishes and ask that they make a special plate of side dishes for you. Stay away from restaurant pasta. Whole-wheat pasta is rare (if non-existent) in restaurants and they all cook pasta with oil. If you're at a steak house, order vegetable side dishes and head straight for the salad bar.

And during holiday gatherings with family and friends, eat before you get there to curb your appetite – and follow the RAVE rules. You'll always be able to find something to eat.

Following the RAVE Diet can be as simple or complicated as you want to make it. If you need recipes, look at the sample recipes in this book and explore the web site recipe links that contain thousands of delicious recipes (See *Part 5 – Recipes On The Web.*) – but leave out any refined or animal foods and use vegetable oil substitutes. (See *Part 4 – Cooking Without Oil.*)

For convenience, use frozen fruits and vegetables. They're almost as good as fresh and may be better in some cases due to modern storage and transportation techniques.

Many people will agree with the health aspects of the RAVE Diet, but simply can't change their eating habits. First of all, everyone already eats plant foods. Rice, potatoes, lettuce, tomatoes, fruits, bread and so forth are all part of our diets and we all eat a wider range of plant foods than we realize, just too little of them. All you have to do is substitute that slice of steak or chicken on your plate – with *more* plant foods. You'll feel full and just as satisfied as you would with your standard American diet.

If you think you "hate" all vegetables, start by simply eating more of the familiar plant foods you do like. There are so many ways to "disguise" the taste of vegetables with seasonings and sauces that this shouldn't be a barrier. (See *Part 4 – Flavorings.*) You just have to get a little creative with your food preparation. If your budget is tight, buy the vegetables that are on sale. Over time, this will automatically increase the variety in your diet. This may be a challenge at first, but read up on how to prepare vegetables in this book and also what they can do for your body, which may make them go down a little easier.

Just as your taste for meat and dairy products was acquired, you can acquire a taste for foods you thought would be impossible to eat. Take bread, for example. If you buy good-tasting whole grain bread in the first place, you should enjoy the taste of the bread by itself, without any high-fat toppings. Try it. You can acquire the clean taste of "plain" bread after just a few slices and you'll come to love it. Some people "hate" the taste of Portobello mushrooms. Trying grilling them with barbeque or A1 steak sauce. They're delicious and a great substitute for hamburgers. And if you absolutely can't stand mushrooms (or another plant food), put them in a food processor, then mix them into a meal.

Your tastes for food will change with this diet and you'll find over time that you prefer the "cleaner" taste of natural foods.

Plant foods are bulky, which means you end up eating more food, in terms of quantity, but you'll actually consume fewer calories. One of the biggest problems is convenience in that you usually won't find healthy, organic food at your local convenience store. This diet does not have to be inconvenient, you just have to think ahead and think in terms of whole plant foods.

Getting More Bang for the Buck

The idea of nutrient density *per calorie*[78] is critical to reversing any disease. Our standard diets are critically deficient in micronutrients, which are vital to restoring and reversing disease. Since we can only eat so many calories, we have to ensure we are getting the biggest nutrient bang for the calorie buck.

When it comes to specific foods, green vegetables are the big winners and densest, per calorie, of any food on the planet. Next are cruciferous vegetables (the cabbage and broccoli family) which are powerful weapons against all forms of cancer.

The following lists the top winners in terms of overall nutrient density:[79]

collards, mustard greens, turnip greens, kale, watercress, bok choy, spinach, Brussels sprouts, swiss chard, arugala, radish, cabbage, bean sprouts, red peppers, romaine lettuce, broccoli, tomatoes, cauliflower, beans

---

[78] You should only compare foods on a per calorie basis because we eat our food based upon calories, rather than weight. It's also the correct way to "normalize" comparisons of foods. If you see any other comparison that is not done on a per calorie basis, the results can be very misleading. The favorite trick by food manufacturers is to compare foods by weight, which is one way they can make a nutritionally bad product look good.

[79] There are many nutrient density lists using slightly different criteria, which show slightly different results. This was based on "Eat Right America" Food Scoring Guide from Dr. Furhmans e-book available at www.drfurhman.com.

The foods shown below should be part of your every day eating plan:

1) Dark leafy green vegetables (avoid iceberg)
2) Solid green vegetables (asparagus, artichokes, celery, cucumber, green peppers, string beans, zucchini)
3) Other vegetables (mushrooms, onions, eggplant, peppers, squash)
4) Cruciferous vegetables (broccoli, cauliflower, watercress)
5) Beans and legumes (red kidney beans, pinto beans, peas, lentils, black-eyes peas, black beans)

See *Part 5 – Food Lists* for a more extensive listing of foods.

Realistically, you will want to eat a wide variety of foods in order to make your meals both high in nutrients, as well as satisfying.

What To Expect

"If this is dying, I highly recommend it." – Bonnie Kramer, who had been pronounced "terminal" by conventional doctors and beat her cancer through nutritional therapy

The body obviously reacts to nutritional therapy much differently than it reacts to toxic treatments like chemo and radiation. Your body will be very happy that you chose this route because it is cleansing and positive in every sense. Remember, the point is to rebuild your entire body, which will serve as the foundation for reversing the root cause of cancer.

How long will it take? That really depends on: 1) how far the cancer has progressed and 2) how damaged your body is. The strategy is to change the biochemistry of your body and rebuild your immune system with diet so it can stem the cancer tide and turn it back, for good.

Dr. Jane Plant,[80] who had breast cancer, suffered through a radical mastectomy, three further operations, 40 radiations treatments, five radiation treatments of her ovaries and 12 chemotherapy treatments. The tumors kept coming back. Not just once or twice, but five times to different parts of her body. The last tumor was on her neck and treatments were not effective. She then changed to a low-fat, plant-based diet and *within days* the lump started to soften and shrink. Within six weeks the tumor was completely gone.

Dr. Plant's success was dramatic and that should not be expected by everyone because there are so many variables involved. But it does demonstrate how effective dietary change can be.

---

[80] The No-Dairy Breast Cancer Prevention Program, Jane Plant.

In other cases, the change can take a different course. We tend to be obsessed with the tumor because it is conventional medicine's target of treatment. Because you are healing *from within*, often the cancer will be gone, but the tumor will remain, even though it has turned non-cancerous. Tumors are most often a mixture of malignant and benign cells and, in fact, most have only a small percentage of cancer cells.

A woman recently wrote to me who had a ping-pong ball sized tumor in her thyroid gland. It had been biopsied and she had received three different medical opinions confirming the cancerous nature of the tumor. She had tried different natural, but non-nutritional therapies and none was working. She then watched the *Healing Cancer From Inside Out* film, and started following the RAVE Diet. Within a week, the Achilles tendonitis she had had for 15 year in both ankles, the arthritis in her left knee and shoulder – which she had had for 10 years – all suddenly disappeared. After two weeks, her heart palpitations ceased, her numerous and "violent" hot flashes were reduced to one mild episode after showering and she started sleeping through the night (she had sleep apnea and used a breathing machine). In addition, she experienced significant weight loss, which her family attributed to the cancer, but she could not believe it because her skin had became more radiant. As she said, "I was only trying to get rid of the cancer!" and yet all these wonderful side-benefits started occurring, one after the next. After several months on the diet, she was re-tested for cancer – and they could not detect any cancer. They removed the tumor for cosmetic reasons, biopsied it, and found not a single malignant cell. As she stated, "I still have my thyroid gland and thus on no drugs or hormones to mimic its function."[81]

In fact, nutritional therapy was rebuilding her body and strengthening it, so her body could fight the cancer – and it won the battle *from inside out*. The point is that recovery times will vary, as there are countless variables involved. It could take anywhere from a month to a year before the cancer is reversed. The only way you will know for sure is by testing for your cancer markers. In the meantime, however, if you are making progress you will notice a host of changes in your body within a few weeks. Appetite returns, pain diminishes, sleep improves and, yes, in almost all cases tumors recede and vanish. Don't be concerned about the tumor as much as the signs that your body is rebuilding and healing itself.

Be warned, however, that the healing process has its ups and downs. A rise in energy may be followed by a sudden downturn. Don't be discouraged as this is typical. Focus on staying on the course you have chosen.

With regard to the diet itself, everyone is different and people will react somewhat differently to any new diet they adopt. Here are just some of the possible experiences you might have when adopting the RAVE Diet.

---

[81] This is from private correspondence. A quote from her letter is currently posted on the www.RaveDiet.com website.

Cravings: Some people experience cravings for some foods, particularly sweets, chocolate and cheese.[82] Hard as this may be to believe, these are withdrawal symptoms that are not totally uncommon when switching to the RAVE Diet. Such foods are actually addictive and food manufacturers have invested heavily in juggling ingredients to make foods as addictive as possible. The problem is that we've lost our taste for real food because most food we eat today is smothered with salt, fat, sweets and chemicals. As a result, our taste buds are currently "warped." It normally takes about three weeks for tastes to change. If you stick with the RAVE Diet, your cravings for the "highs" of sugar, fat and salt will go away as your taste buds return to normal boundaries.

Hunger In-Between Meals: Some people get hungry before lunch, others in mid-afternoon, depending on the meal beforehand. This happens most often with people who are trying to lose weight because they will cut back on portions. This is a mistake on the RAVE Diet because all the foods are low calorie to begin with. Some people will skimp on breakfast and get hungry before noon. Add whole grain products to your breakfast, such as oatmeal, and whole wheat bread. (By the way, oatmeal is *the* most filling breakfast food.) If you eat salads for lunch, make it a meal salad (think big!) and add a handful of beans. Or have a baked sweet potato with it or another side dish. If you're at work, bring your own food and make sure you have enough to snack on if you need to. At dinner, use brown rice or sweet potatoes to fill you up. Don't be afraid to eat because you'll probably consume a larger quantity of food on the RAVE Diet than you did previously – until your body adjusts. The quantity is not as important as the type of foods you're eating.

Constipation Cured: A good bowel movement is one of the most under-appreciated aspects of American life. With the RAVE Diet, your constipation will be cured and, for most, this will be the biggest immediate change. You'll not only experience bowel movements like you've never had them before, but you'll also be getting rid of toxic substances in your body on a regular basis. And if you're accustomed to reading the newspaper while sitting on the toilet, that pastime will be history because you won't have time! Nor, will you experience the straining you used to put up with (which can result in varicose veins). Some people will find they have two to three bowel movements a day (one after every meal). Far from being abnormal, this is actually the ideal. Parenthetically, constipation (and the accompanying straining) is a common side effect of high-protein, low-carb diets. It's not surprising that profits of laxative makers skyrocket when low-carb diets are the craze.[83] Our intent is to put these

---

[82] Many find cheese to be the most difficult food to give up. Part of the reason for this has to do with the casomorphin in cow's milk, which has a subtle addicting and pain-killing quality about it. So yes, Marge, there is morphine in cow's milk. Ever wonder where that chocolate "high" came from?

[83] AP, "Diet Trends May Broaden Demographics," 3/30/04.

businesses out of business because once you've adopted the RAVE Diet, you'll never have to take a laxative again.

Detoxification: What you will be doing on this diet is a natural form of detoxification. Most of us have a lot of toxicity stored within our cellular tissue. As soon as the shift is made to more natural foods, the body will begin to release toxins. Pollutants concentrate in areas of fat tissue, so if you are carrying a lot of fat, toxins will be released when you lose it. The high fiber content of the diet will bind with toxins in your system and take them out away, the same way fiber binds with cholesterol, excess sex hormones and other substances and removes them from your system. A very small percentage of individuals may feel a lack of energy or fatigue initially, as well as other mild side effects. This is the result of the body detoxifying itself. People who quit smoking often experience exactly the same feelings. Stick with it! This will pass as your body gets rid of toxins and adjusts to this new way of eating. Your energy will return and return at a much higher level than before. Other people have experienced headaches. This is similar to withdrawal from caffeine. Again, stick with it. This is a classic sign of detoxification and the headaches or other side effects will go away.

Initial Gas: Due to the high fiber content of the RAVE Diet, you may initially experience more flatulence than normal. As your body transitions to the RAVE Diet, however, that problem will go away and you won't have any more gas than you did on your old diet. A side benefit: The gas from eating plant foods is nowhere near as smelly as the gas you get from eating animal foods (scientific fact). You'll also find that not only your breath, but also your body odor is much sweeter smelling. Parenthetically, refined plant products, such as refined soy and rice products, cause more gas than whole, natural plant foods.

Not Eating Animal Food: Some will, no doubt, experience anxiety because they think they're going to miss an essential nutrient by not eating animal foods. (See *Part 3 – Protein*.) This is a measure of the brainwashing we have all experienced, not only from the meat and dairy industries, but also from our own government, doctors and dieticians. Trust me, only good health will result. This is, after all, the way humans have been eating throughout our history. A neighbor of mine told me that he couldn't sleep without having a slab of steak or chicken before he went to bed. He was clinically obese and still is. *You* won't have any problems sleeping on this diet. In fact, I wish I had a dime for everyone who told me how good he or she felt by *not* eating animals. You will, too, and it will help you sleep more soundly.

Pleasure Traps: We're living in a sea of food advertisements which constantly tell us it's "Ok" to eat bad foods. During holidays, in particular, your friends will encourage you to eat bad foods and it's difficult to resist these temptations. This is the "Pleasure Trap,"[84] and often results in backsliding and moving away from the RAVE Diet altogether. Once you do that, you'll end up

---

[84] For more on this concept, see The Pleasure Trap, Douglas J. Lisle and Alan Goldhamer.

back where you started. Simply stated, the Pleasure Trap means you will be caught in a trap of immediate pleasure, which undermines the long-term goals you have set for yourself. You'll be sacrificing long-term pleasures (conquering cancer, and the lifestyle that goes with that) for the short-term pleasures of high sugar, salt and fatty foods. If you find yourself caught in the Pleasure Trap, here is what I would suggest: Get off the animal and refined foods completely for at least three weeks. The process of withdrawal is not all that different from what one experiences with cigarettes. It takes about three weeks to change your taste buds – roughly the same amount of time it takes a smoker to really feel he or she is over the nicotine hump. And just as cigarettes will always be a lure to a smoker, so too will animal and refined foods to someone who was once addicted to them. Stay away from these foods for at least three weeks and the cravings should come under control, if they're not gone altogether. Find substitutes in herbs, spices and sauces. As your taste buds get used to these flavors, you will come to prefer them. Get smart and follow the RAVE admonition "No Exceptions" – and stick with it. The long-term rewards are far too great to sacrifice for short-term pleasures.

Carbophobia Conquered: You'll be able to enjoy carbohydrates of all varieties – so long as they come from *whole,* natural foods. The carbohydrates you should rightly be afraid of are from refined foods. One misconception about high carbohydrate diets is that they raise triglycerides (blood fats). This is a common misconception based on tests done with *refined* or simple carbohydrates, which *will* raise triglycerides. If you're eating only *complex* carbs found in natural foods, triglyceride levels will not go up. In fact, the best way to dramatically reduce triglycerides is to follow the RAVE Diet – the combination of complex carbohydrates and exercise will reduce triglycerides better than any other approach. (In a few people, who are sensitive, any form of fruit will raise triglycerides because the primary sugar is fructose, a simple sugar.) There is so much confusion about carbohydrates, it would take a book to sort them out. Instead, just remember the refined carbohydrates are the bad guys, while whole food carbs are the good guys.

Sniping Remarks From Uninformed "Friends": In social occasions, I normally do not bring up diet, but if you are eating, it's often inevitable. A remark often heard by people is that low-fat diets are dangerous. This is how strange our attitudes toward food are. The fact we consider a diet that actually reverses heart disease and cancer to be dangerous is nothing short of outrageous! Yet the diet your friends are on – which causes heart disease and cancer – is considered to be safe. The same people who call low-fat diets dangerous are, in fact, eating the most dangerous diet in the world, which kills half the population with cardiovascular disease – and even more through cancer and other diseases. People eating RAVE-like diets are in excellent health throughout the world and a low-fat diet is the healthiest – and safest – diet in the world. There are billions who can attest to that. Unfortunately, very few are Americans and I'm sure very few are your friends.

Better Skin: Because you are clearing out your blood vessels, the blood flow carrying oxygen and nutrients throughout your body will be greatly enhanced and will produce some amazing results. Some people have even had "liver" or "sun spots" disappear from their skin when they adopted this diet. Other people have told me that if they don't consume oils, their skin will dry out. This is a misconception, and a greasy one. Most people have dry skin because they are dehydrated due to their diet. Restrict your consumption of diuretics, which take more fluid out of your body than they bring in – and increase your consumption of plain water and plant foods (which contain high amounts of water). Doing this will keep your skin moist and fresh and do more for your wrinkles than any skin cream on the market. The most common diuretics are coffee, tea and similar stimulants, as well as alcohol.

Better Senses: Largely as a result of opening up your blood vessels, there will be a range of changes you will notice over time, including better hearing, eyesight, taste, smell and touch.

Cheaper Grocery Bill: Many complain about the higher cost of organic foods, but overall, you will save money on groceries. One estimate, made some years ago, pegged the savings at around $1,400 a year. If fruits and vegetables are expensive in your area, use frozen fruits and vegetables instead of fresh. Frozen produce is often packed at the peak of freshness and will also taste better than out-of-season produce. The big savings with the RAVE Diet is not on groceries, however, but current and future health care and medication costs.

Blaming the Diet? Don't blame this diet for coincidental things that may happen to you either physically or mentally. I've heard everything from a man's hair turning gray, to someone's depression blamed on this diet. Don't worry. Your nails, hair and everything else will continue to grow just fine, if not better than ever. The only thing you may experience are anxiety attacks because you think you're not getting enough protein or calcium, especially after you watch the next food advertisement on television. You'll get over it. A year after adopting this diet, you'll have a completely different view of food that will make your doctor smile at your next checkup.

Food Sensitivities/Allergies: In rare cases, the increase in consumption of whole plant foods may trigger food sensitivities or food allergies simply because you're eating more of certain foods. In these cases, it is a matter of finding out which foods are triggers and eliminating them from your diet or cutting back on them. For specific information on a variety of "trigger" foods, get a copy of *Foods That Fight Pain, Neal Barnard, M.D.* A few have experienced gluten intolerance, or Celiac Disease. This is the result of eating more wheat-related foods. The RAVE Diet did not cause the Celiac Disease. You always had an intolerance for gluten (the protein in wheat-related foods) and the diet just brought it out due to increased consumption of wheat. There is a simple solution: Stop eating all forms of wheat (including durum, semolina, spelt, kamut, einkorn and faro) and related grains such as rye, barley and triticale. You can substitute rice, sweet potatoes, etc. or there are gluten-free products that are becoming increasingly available.

Stopping the Diet: This is not the easiest diet to follow, particularly given the social pressures and tempting foods that are all around us. You might think of this as a "temporary" diet designed to fight cancer that can be abandoned once the cancer is under control. Unfortunately, there have been many, many, many cases where people have defeated cancer, abandoned the diet, reintroduced "healthy" chicken and/or fish back into their diets and guess what? The cancer returned.

This is precisely what happened in the famous case of Anthony Sattilaro,[85] an M.D. who contracted a terminal case of prostate cancer. He was given less than a year to live. Quite by accident, he stumbled across the macrobiotic diet. Although skeptical, he adopted the diet and decided to stick with it because of one significant thing, which started happening very soon after he switched his eating habits: *The terrible pain he was suffering started to diminish!* He found he needed less pain medication and *in just three weeks* his cancer pain was completely gone. His energy came back and he was able to return to work. A year later, he was re-tested for cancer and it was completely gone. He remained cancer-free for ten years – until he reintroduced chicken and fish into his diet. Despite ten years of being declared free of cancer after his change in diet, his medical mind was still not totally convinced the diet had made the difference although, paradoxically, he did admit his change in diet brought the cancer back. Despite this, he continued eating chicken and fish and he was soon on narcotic painkillers – until the cancer killed him.

A woman contracted breast cancer and cured it by using natural treatments and adopting a plant-based diet.[86] Years after her cancer was gone – thinking she was somehow immune from cancer – she decided to return to her previous diet – which included "healthy" chicken and fish. Just like Dr. Sattilaro, soon after she changed back to her old diet, she contracted breast cancer for the second time. Unlike Dr. Sattilaro, however, she switched back to a RAVE-like diet and underwent natural treatments for a second time. Fortunately, her breast cancer vanished once again. She had learned her lesson about the power of diet for the last time.

These are just two stories, but there are many more which illustrate that you have to permanently change your diet and lifestyle if you want to keep cancer (and other diseases) out of your body.

---

[85] He wrote a book about the experience called Recalled By Life, Anthony Satillaro.
[86] Triumph Over Cancer, Agi Lidle.

Supplementation

You cannot put nature in a pill.

People love their supplements, almost as much as they hate their vegetables. What most are trying to do is make up for their bad eating habits, but that is simply not possible because isolated synthetic supplements are weak substitutes for the vibrant strength of the integrated micronutrients you get from whole plant foods in their natural states. For example, a few years back, there was a study that showed taking supplements containing lycopene from tomatoes, did *nothing* to lower the risk of prostate cancer, whereas natural whole tomatoes, containing an integrated, complex profile of nutrients, did lower the risk.[87]

Remember when vitamin C was the rage? Everyone was taking vitamin C tablets like they were going out of style. Then it was discovered that vitamin C wasn't very well absorbed unless a couple of bioflavonoids were present (hesperidin and rutin). So the manufacturers re-tooled and added these bioflavonoids to the pills and everything was supposed to be Ok again. Except it was later discovered that despite the presence of these bioflavonoids, the body couldn't absorb vitamin C very well unless calcium was present as well. So the pills were re-formulated with bioflavonoids *and* calcium. So, while the public remained confused – but, nonetheless, kept swallowing their vitamin C tablets – they continued to overlook a source of vitamin C that had *all* the elements together and allowed optimal absorption of the vitamin: citrus fruits, such as oranges and grapefruits, as well as most other plant foods. While scientists were baffled trying to come up with one or two or three key ingredients that would allow the body to effectively absorb vitamin C in pill form, people forgot that nature had already come up with a solution to this problem in the form of whole plant foods, which contain thousands of nutrient profiles that scientists are still in the dark about.[88] This is borne out by the fact that just a small glass of orange juice containing only 37 mg of vitamin C is twice as likely to lower the risk of stomach cancer as 1,000 mg of vitamin C in pill form.

When you peruse the newspapers, you'll see reports of studies which show that this vitamin or that vitamin had no effect on combating a particular disease. What you have to pay attention to is that always – without exception – these studies are looking at the synthetic version of the vitamin – a pill – which has no magic. There's no mojo in a pill. What you will never see is a study which states that a vitamin taken in its natural state had no effect on a disease. Natural vitamins found in food always have a positive effect!

---

[87] Tomatoes May Be Better Against Cancer Than Lycopene Alone, LA Times, 11/10/03.
[88] Lessons From the Miracle Doctors, Jon Barron, p. 54

A well-reported study found that beta-carotene *supplements* actually *increasing* the risk of lung cancer in heavy smokers.[89] It's also been found that vitamin A or beta-carotene supplements may also interfere with the absorption of carotenoids such as lutein and lycopene, and this interference can increase the risks of developing cancer.[90] You will never find this to be the case with natural sources of beta-carotene found in food.

Recently it was reported that after spending millions of dollars, scientists found that vitamins E and selenium *synthetic supplements* were useless for combating prostate cancer.[91] A number of other recent studies using synthetic supplements came to the same conclusion.[92] Supplements alone won't make a dent against cancer. You have to change your overall diet and lifestyle. Supplements may help, but taking them alone without changing your diet and lifestyle won't blow the cancer candle out!

The findings of such studies are not surprising because synthetic supplements – concentrated and *isolated* forms of vitamins and minerals – throw the body off balance because nowhere can such concentrations be found in nature. And *the body has been trained to expect what comes from nature.*

People always assume that more is better. When it comes to supplements, however, that is usually not the case. Vitamin A supplements have been shown to cause a one in 57 chance of birth defects when taken by pregnant women, as well as increasing the risk of hip fractures in older women.[93] Iron supplementation has been shown to cause a fatal liver disease.[94] Magnesium supplementation has been shown to increase the risk of heart attacks and sudden death, particularly among

---

[89] The effect of vitamin E and beta carotene on the incidence of lung cancer and other cancers in male smokers, The Alpha-Tocopherol, Beta Carotene Cancer Prevention Study Group, NEJM, 1994 Apr 14;330(15):1029-35; Omenn GS, Effects of a combination of beta carotene and vitamin A on lung cancer and cardiovascular disease, N Engl J Med. 1996 May 2;334(18):1150-5.

[90] Mayne ST. Beta-carotene, carotenoids, and disease prevention in humans. FASEB. 1996;10(7):690-701.

[91] See The SELECT Prostate Cancer Prevention Trial at http://www.cancer.gov/clinicaltrials/digestpage/SELECT

[92] Jennifer Lin, et al., Vitamins C and E and Beta Carotene Supplementation and Cancer Risk: A Randomized Controlled Trial. J. Natl. Cancer Inst..2008; 0: djn438 v1-23; Vitamins C and E and Beta Carotene Again Fail to Reduce Cancer Risk in Randomized Controlled Trial. J Natl Cancer Inst 2008 0: djn501v1-1.

[93] Michaelsson K., Serum retinol levels and the risk of fracture, N Engl J Med. 2003 Jan 23;348(4):287-94; Dolk HM, Dietary vitamin A and teratogenic risk: European Teratology Society discussion paper, Eur J Obstet Gynecol Reprod Biol. 1999 Mar;83(1):31-6; Rothman KJ. Teratogenicity of high vitamin A intake. N Engl J Med. 1995 Nov 23;333(21):1369-73.

[94] Schumann K., Safety aspects of iron in food, Ann Nutr Metab. 2001;45(3):91-101.

people with heart disease.[95] Zinc *and* iron supplements may also increase the risk of death from heart disease.[96]

Folic acid supplementation has been shown to reduce the risk of birth defects, but it was recently discovered it also increased the risks of colon cancer.[97] It's been found that getting enough folic acid may keep tumors from starting up by repairing DNA errors, but getting too much may feed tumors once they start.[98]

There is also controversy about taking synthetic antioxidant supplementation during radiation treatments with reports showing they interfered with the treatment's "effectiveness."[99] Although the dust is still settling on this controversy, what is clear is that the adverse reactions were only experienced by those who still smoked. But the bottom line is that the micronutrients from whole foods will *always* help, even with smokers.

The examples are really endless and they all point to the same thing: Artificial, synthetic supplements throw the body off balance and can result in serious and unexpected side effects. Natural foods in their natural packages keep the body in balance.

You will no doubt run across testimonials regarding initial positive results from taking many supplements (from herbal extracts to mango juice and so on). If true, these can be ascribed to the placebo effect. Over the long-term, however, it has not been shown that supplements work against cancer – unless you take care of the fundamentals of diet and lifestyle. That is to say, if you take wonder supplement #1 and you're eating hamburgers all day, that supplement may make

---

[95] Galloe AM, Influence of oral magnesium supplementation on cardiac events among survivors of an acute myocardial infarction, BMJ, 1993 Sep 4;307(6904):585-7.

[96] Galloe AM, Influence of oral magnesium supplementation on cardiac events among survivors of an acute myocardial infarction, BMJ, 1993 Sep 4;307(6904):585-7; Black MR, Zinc supplements and serum lipids in young adult white males, Am J Clin Nutr. 1988 Jun;47(6):970-5.

[97] See Fortifying foods with the vitamin has reduced certain birth defects but may have raised rates of colon cancer, Los Angeles Times, August 6, 2007.

[98] Ulrich C., Folate and cancer prevention: a closer look at a complex picture, Am J Clin Nut; 2007; 86(2)271-273.

[99] Bairati I, Meyer F, Jobin E, Gélinas M, Fortin A, Nabid A, Brochet F, Têtu B., Antioxidant vitamins supplementation and mortality: a randomized trial in head and neck cancer patients, Int J Cancer. 2006;119(9):2221-4; Lawenda B et al. Should supplemental antioxidant administration be avoided during chemotherapy and radiation therapy?, J Natl Canc Inst. 2008;100:773–783; Meyer F, Bairati I, Jobin E, Gélinas M, Fortin A, Nabid A, Têtu B., Acute adverse effects of radiation therapy and local recurrence in relation to dietary and plasma beta carotene and alpha tocopherol in head and neck cancer patients., Nutr Cancer. 2007;59(1):29-35; Meyer F, Bairati I, Fortin A, Gélinas M, Nabid A, Brochet F, Têtu B., Interaction between antioxidant vitamin supplementation and cigarette smoking during radiation therapy in relation to long-term effects on recurrence and mortality: a randomized trial among head and neck cancer patients. Int J Cancer. 2008;122(7):1679-83.

you feel much better (despite the hamburgers), but once the placebo effect wears off, you will come crashing down with the reality of your diet.[100]

Synthetic supplements have their place in deficiency diseases, such as scurvy, which is caused by a deficiency of vitamin C. But cancer is not a deficiency disease of a single nutrient[101] and cannot be healed with the application of a single or even multiple nutrients, particularly in synthetic form. A vitamin's benefit, in other words, will become apparent only if people are not getting enough of it. Supplementation can have a place in the short-term healing of diseases, but in the long-term, they will cause problems.

With regard to short-term supplementation, if you are currently undergoing conventional treatments you will no doubt need supplementation of some sort because of the devastating effects of chemo on the body. However, many of the most common herbal supplements have the potential to interact with cancer drugs in negative ways, so you need to tell your oncologist about what you are doing.[102] You should also seek advice about supplements from a clinic which has experience using them with people who are either currently undergoing conventional treatments or have undergone such treatments.

To be sure, we have nutritional deficiencies in the area of micronutrients, particularly those that fight cancer, but our bodies work as a symphony and the absorption of micronutrients from whole plant foods will orchestrate the healing of the body in a way that single or multiple magic bullet supplements cannot.

Combined with a good anti-cancer diet, natural, non-toxic supplementation can play a role in helping heal cancer. This book is about creating the foundation for healing cancer through nutrition and there are simply too many supplements out there to evaluate thoroughly, so I would encourage you to investigate them on your own. I will discuss a few methods of natural supplementation, below.

Green Juicing and Blending

The primary form of dietary supplementation on this diet is in the form of green juicing because it is a way of getting highly concentrated nutrients from high-nutrient plant foods into your system. Consult the *Green Juicing* section

---

[100] One example of a wonder supplement not working by itself is a lady with cancer who was supplementing her typical American diet with Hoxey's herbal tonic. It had no effect whatsoever. As soon as she changed to the RAVE Diet, however, she noticed beneficial results and within six months, had reversed her cancer. Hoxey's tonic can be a good supplement, but the odds of it reversing cancer by itself are pretty long.

[101] Proponents of laetrile will argue that cancer is caused by a deficiency of vitamin B-17, but B-17 supplementation is neither the cause nor the cure for cancer. For more discussion on laetrile, see *Supplementation – Laetrile*.

[102] In one study, researchers found that nearly half of women being treated for breast and gynecologic cancers used some type of herbal or vitamin supplement and of those, half did not inform their doctors. See Journal of Clinical Oncology Vol. 22, No. 4: 671-677.

under *Sample Recipes* for a variety of recipes. If you do not have a juicer or cannot afford one, you can take the recipes to a local juice bar and they can make them for you. Be sure to call to make sure they have the right ingredients. It's important that you drink the juice right after it is made because it will lose much of its potency if you have it sit around too long.

I would recommend that you consume juiced drinks on an occasional basis, in addition to your regular meals. It is an optional component of the diet.

Wheatgrass is also an excellent dietary supplement. Again, you can have it juiced for you at most natural foods markets and juice bars. It is very strong-smelling due to the chlorophyll, but goes down easier than it smells. Until you get used to it, take an ounce a day, then increase that to two ounces a day. If you want to grow and juice your own wheatgrass, there are resources on the Internet that can help you.[103] Health clinics which treat cancer patients swear by wheatgrass as a dietary supplement and it has been used for well over 30 years.[104] And a number of recent scientific studies are starting to bear out these claims.[105] Women who are pregnant or breast feeding should not use wheatgrass.

With seriously ill patients who are unable to eat much, juicing can be life-saving as it may be the only way to get a constant supply of nutrients into their bodies.

Ann Wigmore is the woman who introduced wheatgrass to the world and she reversed her own cancer using a natural foods diet with supplementation – after doctors had declared her terminal.

Although she was big on juicing, later in her life she was turning against it and leaning more toward blending because juicing is not the way food is found in nature. The primary problem with juicing is that it leaves most of the fiber in the food behind and fiber is critical to not only fighting cancer, but also any other disease.

---

[103] A good place to start: www.sproutman.com.

[104] See The Wheatgrass Book, Ann Wigmore.

[105] Shyam R et al., Wheat grass supplementation decreases oxidative stress in healthy subjects: a comparative study with spirulina [letter to the editor]. J Altern Complement Med. 13(8):789-791; Marsili V, Calzuola I, Gianfranceschi GL, Nutritional relevance of wheat sprouts containing high levels of organic phosphates and antioxidant compounds. J Clin Gastroenterol. 2004 Jul;38(6 Suppl):S123-6; Peryt B et al., Mechanism of antimutagenicity of wheat sprout extracts. Mutat Res. 269(2):201-215; Bar-Sela G, Tsalic M, Fried G, Goldberg H, Wheat grass juice may improve hematological toxicity related to chemotherapy in breast cancer patients: a pilot study. Nutr Cancer. 58(1):43-8; Marawaha RK et al., Wheat grass juice reduces transfusion requirement in patients with thalassemia major: a pilot study. Indian Pediatr.41(7):716-20; Fernandes CJ & O'Donovan DJ, Natural antioxidant therapy for patients with hemolyticanemia. Indian Pediatr. 42: 618-619; Pole SN, Wheat grass juice in thalassemia. Indian Pediatr. 43(1):79-80; Ben-Arye E et al., Wheat grass juice in the treatment of active distal ulcerative colitis: a randomized double-blind placebo-controlled trial. Scand J Gastroenterol. 37(4):444-449.

This is the reason we refer to juicing as optional supplementation. There are clinics which use nothing but juicing when treating cancer patients and they have had success. I would argue, however, that their success rates would be much higher if they used juicing as a supplement, not the main course.[106]

Unlike juicing, blending includes the whole food, as nothing is left behind. In fact, blending can be part of your every day diet and is an excellent way to get more green vegetables into your meals. Because green blending is very concentrated, you need to add small amounts of semi-sweet vegetables to them, such as carrots or tomatoes, in order to make them more palatable. Consult the *Blending* section under *Sample Recipes* for a variety of recipes.

Vitamin D

If there is a single micronutrient that practically all Americans are deficient in it is vitamin D, known as the "sunshine" vitamin – and having adequate amount of this vitamin is critical in fighting cancer.[107]

Because of our lifestyles, we simply do not get out in the sun much, which accounts for the deficiency. Of course, there are vitamin D supplements but, they cannot hold a candle to the "supercharged" vitamin D you can get naturally.

Unfortunately, sun screens block the production of vitamin D, so you have to get a little sunlight *before* you put on sunscreen. Also, you should allow full-spectrum sunlight to enter your eyes, so avoid wearing sunglasses.

Here are some general rules of thumb: During the summer, from 10 a.m. to 2 p.m. (the angle of the sun is important), fair-skinned people should get just 10 minutes of exposure, while very dark-skinned people should get 30 minutes, several times a week. Those with skin colors in-between can adjust accordingly. You should expose about 25% of your body, i.e., face, hands and arms or arms and legs. Use your common sense and never, ever allow yourself to come close to being sunburned. In fact, if you know how long it will take before you burn, about one-quarter of that time would be adequate. Moderate sunlight exposure during the summer is enough to allow you to maintain healthy vitamin D levels throughout the year because the body stores this vitamin and releases it as needed.

---

[106] Of course, if juicing is the only way to get nutrients into someone, because of their condition, then juicing will have the main role.

[107] Grant WB. An estimate of premature cancer mortality in the U.S. due to inadequate doses of solar ultraviolet-B radiation. Cancer 2002;94:1867-75; Hanchette CL and Schwartz GG. Geographic patterns of prostate cancer mortality. Evidence for a protective effect of ultraviolet radiation. Cancer 1992;70:2861-9. Note that vitamin D has receptors in more than 36 organs throughout the body, which means a deficiency of this vitamin will impact your fight against cancer.

If you cannot get out in the sun, especially in the winter months, the recommended supplement dosage should be 1,000 IU a day.[108] The government has set the safe upper limit at 2,000 IU a day.[109]

Despite the bad publicity regarding indoor tanning facilities, they can be safe if used responsibly and – most importantly – the facility uses low-pressure lamps, which emit a balance of UVA and UVB rays.

Because of the PR job done by institutions such as the American Cancer Society, many people are practically hysterical about exposing their skin to the sun for fear of getting skin cancer – despite the fact humans have a biological need to get this vitamin from the sun! The current hysteria is not justified and can actually do severe damage to your health. For example, the highest rates of melanoma, the most deadly skin cancer, are found in people who spend most of their time indoors away from the sun, and melanomas usually occur in parts of the body that receive no sun exposure. In addition, there is no credible scientific evidence that moderate sun exposure causes melanomas.[110] In fact, there are many scientific studies showing a lower incidence of melanoma when people are regularly exposed to sunlight.[111] People who received a lot of sun exposure up to the time of their melanoma diagnosis had better survival rates than those who received little sun exposure.[112]

Keep in mind that when we get sunburned, the redness is caused by blood rushing to the skin in order to repair damaged cells and destroy any that have turned cancerous. If your immune system is running on empty, the repair job will be less than perfect, leaving cancer cells behind to multiply – which goes a long way in explaining why we have a skin cancer epidemic in this country, despite spending less time outdoors than our forebears. With a strong immune system, there won't be a problem. In fact, squamous cell and basel cell cancers should easily go away with this diet.

---

[108] Taken from The UV Advantage, Michael F. Holick, Ph.D., p. 150. Vitamin D recommendations vary widely. And as our knowledge increases about this vitamin, the recommended dosage goes up. See also, Wolpowitz D, Gilchrest BA., The vitamin D questions: how much do you need and how should you get it? J Am Acad Dermatol. 2006 Feb;54(2):301-17; Reichrath J, The challenge resulting from positive and negative effects of sunlight: how much solar UV exposure is appropriate to balance between risks of vitamin D deficiency and skin cancer? Prog Biophys Mol Biol. 2006 Sep;92(1):9-16; Vieth R. What is the optimal vitamin D status for health? Prog Biophys Mol Biol. 2006 Sep;92(1):26-32.

[109] Taken from the Harvard Medical School Family Guide. See www.health.harvard.edu/fhg/updates/update0204a.shtml

[110] The UV Advantage, Michael F. Holick, Ph.D., p. 14.

[111] Berwick M, Armstrong BK, Ben-Porat L, et al., Sun exposure and mortality from melanoma. J Natl Cancer Inst. 2005;97:195-199; Millen AE, Tucker MA, Hartge P, et al., Diet and melanoma in a case-control study. Cancer Epidemiol Biomarkers Prev. 2004;13:1042-1051.

[112] Berwick M, Armstrong BK, Ben-Porat L, et al., Sun exposure and mortality from melanoma. J Natl Cancer Inst. 2005;97:195-199.

The consumption of animal protein has a tendency to block the production of the vitamin D we receive from the sun, thereby reducing the amount of "supercharged" vitamin D available to our bodies.[113] This is just another reason to eliminate animal products from our diets. Bottom line? A good diet can do more to thwart skin cancer than staying away from the sun. Sun exposure should be encouraged because the benefits for cancer prevention[114] and reversal are incalculable.

Vitamin C

Vitamin C has long been known to be effective against cancer not only because it's an antioxidant, which can handle free radicals, but it can also selectively destroy cancer cells without harming healthy cells.[115] Clinics throughout the world[116] have been using high-dose *intravenous* vitamin C with success and recent studies[117] have confirmed the value of IV C. It would be worth you investigation to find out if this treatment is right for you.

---

[113] The China Study, T. Colin Campbell, Ph.D., p. 180.

[114] Holick MF, Vitamin D: importance in the prevention of cancers, type 1 diabetes, heart disease, and osteoporosis. Am J Clin Nutr. 2004 Mar;79(3):362-71; Robsahm TE, Tretli S, Dahlback A, Moan J, Vitamin D3 from sunlight may improve the prognosis of breast-, colon- and prostate cancer (Norway), Cancer Causes Control. 2004 Mar;15(2):149-58; Zhou W, Suk R, et al., Vitamin D is associated with improved survival in early-stage non-small cell lung cancer patients, Cancer Epidemiol Biomarkers Prev. 2005 Oct;14(10):2303-9; Berwick M, Armstrong BK, et al., Sun exposure and mortality from melanoma, J Natl Cancer Inst. 2005 Feb 2;97(3):195-9.

[115] Chen Q, et al., Pharmacologic doses of ascorbate act as a pro-oxidant and decrease growth of aggressive tumor xenografts in mice. Proceedings of the National Academy of Sciences 2008; 105:11105–11109; Frei B, et al., Vitamin C and cancer revisited. Proceedings of the National Academy of Sciences 2008; 105(32): 11037–11038; Cameron E, et al., The orthomolecular treatment of cancer. II. Clinical trial of high-dose ascorbic acid supplements in advanced human cancer. Chemico-Biological Interactions 1974; 9:285–315; Cameron E, et al., Supplemental ascorbate in the supportive treatment of cancer: Prolongation of survival times in terminal human cancer. Proceedings of the National Academy of Sciences 1976; 73:3685–3689; Cameron E, et al., Supplemental ascorbate in the supportive treatment of cancer: Reevaluation of prolongation of survival times in terminal human cancer. 1978; Proceedings of the National Academy of Sciences USA 75:4538–4542.

[116] One such clinic is An Oasis of Hope Hospital, run by Francisco Contreras, M.D. The hospital has treated over 100,000 cancer patients. Their web page: www.oasisofhope.com

[117] Frei B, Lawson S. Vitamin C and cancer revisited. PNAS. 2008;105:11037-11038; Chen Q, Espey MG, Sun AY, Pooput C, Kirk KL, Krishna MC, Khosh DB, Drisko J, Levine M. Pharmacologic doses of ascorbate act as a prooxidant and decrease growth of aggressive tumor xenografts in mice. PNAS. 2008;105:11105-11109.

d be pointed out that there have been numerous "studies" which have
that vitamin C supplements interfere with the effectiveness of
onal treatments.[118] The problem with these studies is that they used an
priate animal: mice. Unlike humans, *mice make their own vitamin C*. In
fact, hen adjusted for body weight, mice synthesize the human body weight
equivalent of approximately 10,000 milligrams of vitamin C each day,[119] which
just might explain why they found a problem with vitamin C supplementation.
Had the researchers used an animal which does not produce their own vitamin C,
such as a human, the results just might have been very different.

Laetrile

Laetrile (amygdalin) – or vitamin B-17 – is without question the most
controversial supplement due to its colorful history. Proponents of laetrile will
argue that cancer is caused by a deficiency of B-17.[120] Given the state of the
Western diet, there is no doubt a B-17 deficiency, but doctors who actually use
laetrile in healing cancer[121] will tell you that diet, not laetrile, is the foundation
for reversing the disease. While laetrile can certainly help, B-17 deficiency is
neither the cause nor is supplementation the cure for cancer.

Dr. Benzil, who had great success reversing cancers for many years using
laetrile with diet, stated it this way:[122]

> *"Laetrile was not a miracle drug or a cancer vitamin or a cancer
> cure, but was just a small part of a total nutritional program."*

Laetrile's claim to fame is that it helps with tumor reduction. In studies with
mice at Sloan-Kettering Hospital, Dr. Kanematsu Suiura's work showed a
remarkable success rate using laetrile treatments, with consistent 75 percent
regressions in experimental animals.[123] Since laetrile is a natural substance and
cannot be patented (and therefore cannot produce big pay days), the cancer
industry was quick to pounce on these findings and discredit Suiura's work.
Sloan-Kettering ran a series of bogus tests which altered Dr. Suiura's protocols

---

[118] Doheny K. Vitamin C and chemotherapy: bad combo? Supplementing with vitamin C
may reduce effectiveness of chemotherapy drugs, study shows. WebMD Health News.
For a good critique of such studies, see www.weeksmd.com/?p=1213.
[119] Chatterjee IB, Majumder AK, Nandi BK, Subramanian N. Synthesis and some major
functions of vitamin C in animals. Ann N Y Acad Sci. 1975 Sep 30;258:24-47.
[120] World Without Cancer: The Story of Vitamin B17, G. Edward Griffin.
[121] See, for example, Alive and Well: One Doctor's Experience with Nutrition in the
Treatment of Cancer Patients, Philip E. Binzel, Jr., M.D.
[122] Alive and Well, Philip E. Binzel, Jr., M.D., pp. 78-79.
[123] The Cancer Industry, Ralph Moss, Ph.D., p. 145.

and – big surprise! – laetrile was found to be *ineffective*. Ralph Moss, who was employed by Sloan-Kettering at the time and a witness to this travesty, blew the whistle on these tests. He was fired the next day. Here is what he said:[124]

> *"Over the course of the next three and a half years, I watched as my employers just lied about the outcome of Dr. Suiura's work, and about what had actually been achieved at Memorial with the laetrile experiments."*

When Dr. Suiura, himself, finally spoke out about this charade, he was fired, as well. So much for the pursuit of truth in the cancer industry!

While tumor reduction is a notable accomplishment – particularly using a natural substance – it is, nonetheless, reduction of a symptom of cancer and this is why the use of laetrile[125] has to be considered as supplementary to the foundation for reversing cancer: diet. Just as you might achieve tumor reduction with radiation and chemotherapy, if you don't address the underlying cause of the tumor, it will return.

While most people may suffer from a B-17 deficiency, it can be easily corrected with the right diet. Laetrile can be found in plant foods such as chick-peas, lentils, lima beans, mung bean sprouts, cashews, alfalfa, barley, brown rice, millet and many more. While over 1,200 different plants contain laetrile, for commercial purposes, it is derived from the kernels of the apricot, peach and the bitter almond.

---

[124] The most complete account of the bogus laetrile testing can be found in The Cancer Industry, Ralph Moss, Ph.D., chapter 9.

[125] More recent successes with food-derived extracts of amygdalin show it effectively kills cancer cells and causes apoptosis in experimental systems. See: Syrigos KN, Rowlinson-Busza G, Epenetos AA, In vitro cytotoxicity following specific activation of amygdalin by beta-glucosidase conjugated to a bladder cancer-associated monoclonal antibody. Int J Cancer. 1998;78:712-9; Kwon HY, Hong SP, Hahn DH, Kim JH, Apoptosis induction of Persicae Semen extract in human promyelocytic leukemia (HL-60) cells. Arch Pharm Res. 2003;26:157-61; Fukuda T, Ito H, Mukainaka T, et al., Anti-tumor promoting effect of glycosides from Prunus persica seeds. Biol Pharm Bull. 2003;26:271-3; Kerr JF, Wyllie AH, Currie AR, Apoptosis: a basic biological phenomenon with wide-ranging implications in tissue kinetics. Br J Cancer. 1972 Aug;26(4):239-57.

Notes

Genetics

"Genes load the gun. Lifestyle pulls the trigger." – Caldwell Esselstyn, M.D.

Although genetic links to cancer only represent a very small fraction of all cancers and the genes-cancer link has been greatly exaggerated (more on this below), it will be covered here 1) because many people incorrectly blame their cancer on their genes; and 2) the risks for people whose genes *are* linked to cancer can be drastically reduced by making simple diet and lifestyle changes, like those contained in this book.

Virtually everyone who is diagnosed with cancer thinks they are eating a healthy diet and living a healthy lifestyle. This is reinforced by misinformed articles in the press, by doctors, and by cancer organizations. Yet the fact that people come down with cancer in the first place should be proof they are neither eating well nor living a healthy life. Because of the misinformation people have in their heads, they start looking at other things, such as genes and environmental pollutants as the cause of their cancer.

We are all born with a matrix of genes which can make us more or less susceptible to a wide range of diseases. The "bad" genes, however, are almost always dormant and do not become active players unless the right conditions set them off. And a bad diet and lifestyle will create those conditions. A healthy diet and lifestyle will keep bad genes quiet and they will never trigger a disease.

There are also people who like to credit their good genes for their health. The Okinawans, for example, are known to have the longest disability-free life expectancy of any people in the world and many Okinawans like to give credit to their genetic makeup. Yet, all you have to do is look at younger Okinawans living near American military bases to shatter that myth. Unlike their parents, Okinawan youth have adopted the American fast food culture and as a result, they have Japan's highest rates of obesity, heart disease and premature death. Also, when Okinawans migrate to America and adopt the American diet and lifestyle, their rates of disease and longevity soon match the American rates.

Most people see genes as immutable and unchanging – you're either doomed or saved by your genetic makeup. This is not at all true and diet and lifestyle can directly affect how your genes are expressed.[126]

---

[126] This is called nutrigenomics. For more information, see "Nutrigenomics in public health nutrition: short-term perspectives", Chavez A, Munoz de Chavez M, European Journal of Clinical Nutrition. 57(Suppl. 1)97-100; "Nutrigenomics: Goals and Perspectives.", Müller M, Kersten S., Nature Reviews Genetics 4. 315 -322; "Nutritional genomics-"Nutrigenomics", Trayhurn P., British Journal Nutrition. 89:1-2.

Dr. Dean Ornish took a small group of men with early stage prostate cancer and put them on a plant-based diet, coupled with exercise. In just three months, the men had changes in activity in about 500 genes, including 48 that were turned on by the diet – and 452 that were turned off![127]

Cigarette smoking changes the expression of genes in cells lining the airways. Some 97 genes were expressed differently than in people who had never smoked.[128]

A gene for a protein that regulates cholesterol is potentially lethal for some smokers, in terms of heart disease. But if they gave up smoking and changed to a healthy diet and lifestyle, their genetic predisposition for heart disease can be completely eliminated.[129]

Women with the BRCA1 and BRCA2 genes have up to an 80 percent risk of developing breast cancer *if* they have a strong family history of breast cancer. Women carrying these genes who do not have a strong family history have only a ten percent chance of developing breast cancer – or about the same as if they didn't have the bad gene at all. That's a whopping 800 percent variation in outcome – all depending on family history. What does family history mean? It means a history of diet and lifestyle that awakens these genes.

That diet and lifestyle have a huge impact can be seen in the fact that women carrying the mutated BRCA1 gene are 60 percent less likely to have breast cancer if they were breast fed for more than a year.[130] It's also been found that women carrying these genes can reduce their risks of breast cancer by up to 65 percent simply by losing weight (regardless of breast feeding).[131] Conversely, it's been found that gaining 10 pounds increased their risk of developing cancer. If you start putting all the healthy diet and lifestyle factors together, you can put these genes to sleep forever.

Even without this bad gene, women who have a family history of breast cancer feel hopeless and are opting for double mastectomies as a prophylactic measure. What they don't realize is that having both breasts removed does not reduce their risks of getting uterine cancer, liver cancer, lymph cancer or a host of other cancers. And there are better ways to reduce their risks of getting breast cancer, regardless of family history.

The latest theory regarding colon cancer is that it's one of the most commonly inherited cancer syndromes known, and the medical intelligentsia has developed an elaborate explanation for this so-called genetically-based disease. What they fail to mention in their explanation is that colon cancer was virtually unknown 100 years ago, and yet it's now the single leading cancer in men and women

---

[127] As reported in MSNBC, June 16, 2008; www.msnbc.msn.com/id/25199024/.
[128] Avrum Spira, et al. Effects of cigarette smoke on the human airway epithelial cell transcriptome. PNAS July 6, 2004 vol. 101 no. 27 10143-10148.
[129] As reported by Ann Underwood, Jerry Adler. Diet and Genes. Newsweek. 1/24/05.
[130] Journal of the National Cancer Institute, July 21, 2004.
[131] As reported by the BBC, August 19, 2005.

combined. Genes don't change across generations in the short span of 100 years. Only diet and lifestyle change that rapidly.

A recent study[132] has shown that genetic links to cancers have been greatly exaggerated and, in fact, genetics is far less important to cancer than past studies (and headlines) have led people to believe. The study analyzed hundreds of other studies that claimed to have discovered genes that cause cancer. It found out that of 240 claimed associations between genes and cancer risk, in fact only two genes actually had any significant correlation at all.[133] That's less than one percent! Another recent study found that genetic testing for heart disease was completely useless.[134] Traditional risk factors, such as smoking, blood pressure and measures of systemic inflammation, were far better predictors of heart disease. In other words, it's not the genetic predisposition that will give you heart disease (or cancer), but your diet and lifestyle.

Another problem with these studies are the words "association" and "correlation" because these are statistical artifacts which do not, in fact, show causation – they in no way show that a specific gene or genes will cause cancer. What does all this mean? Past studies which drew correlations between genetics and cancer exaggerated the significance of such correlations. Why? In my opinion, it was probably an attempt to elevate the importance of genes in the hope of getting research money because drug companies are targeting gene therapy as the new frontier for developing magic bullet drugs. They can then show success with these drugs by using relative (rubber) numbers. The same gene-disease link exaggeration is now happening across the board with other diseases, e.g., Alzheimer's[135] as pharmaceutical companies prepare for a new era of gene-targeted drugs. And profits.

The problem, of course, is that magic bullet treatments have never been successful in treating cancer – or any other degenerative disease – and never will be, due to the nature of these diseases.

If genes were that important, we would simply not have the explosion of diseases that characterizes the American health landscape, i.e., genetic makeup did not create the mess we're in today. Many people are genetically susceptible to adult-onset diabetes, for example. If they eat a diet full of animal and refined foods, it is a virtual certainty they will get diabetes. If they do not eat these foods, they simply will not get diabetes, regardless of their genes. In fact, all

---

[132] As reported in "Many studies needed to tie genes to cancer," Reuters, 12/30/08. See, Zeggini E, Ioannidis JP. Meta-analysis in genome-wide association studies. Pharmacogenomics. 2009 Feb;10(2):191-201.

[133] The study did not examine the BRCA1 or BRCA2 genetic link.

[134] Nina P. Paynter, PhD, et al. Cardiovascular Disease Risk Prediction With and Without Knowledge of Genetic Variation at Chromosome 9p21.3. Annals of Internal Medicine. Vol. 150, 2, pp. 65-72 (20 January 2009).

[135] Kavvoura FK, et al. Evaluation of the potential excess of statistically significant findings in published genetic association studies: application to Alzheimer's disease. Am J Epidemiol. 2008 Oct 15;168(8):855-65.

populations have people within them who are genetically predisposed to certain diseases. But some populations never get these diseases due to their diet and lifestyle. So despite these predispositions, you can overcome genetic weaknesses through diet and lifestyle. And if you never ate these harmful foods, you would never even know about your genetic predispositions. Heart disease and our common cancers were unknown in many countries throughout the world – until the American diet was introduced to them.

Bottom line? Don't count on grandpa's genes to save you from a self-destructive lifestyle. Most of us have nutritional time bombs ticking inside of us. If you're smart, you'll play the odds and change your diet to improve the quality of your life so you can, in fact, grow old gracefully, with dignity, and without a regimen of debilitating drugs.

Environmental Factors

"We are all so contaminated that if we were cannibals our meat would be banned from human consumption." – Paula Baillie-Hamilton, M.D.

It is now possible to detect over 600 different chemicals in our bodies that were not present in any human being before the early 1900s. The Centers for Disease Control recently estimated that the average person has 116 different toxins in their bodies.[136] Drinking water in the U.S. currently contains over 2,100 toxic chemicals that are known to cause cancer, cell mutation and nervous disorders in animals. This shouldn't be surprising considering there are close to 100,000 chemicals now in everyday use with over 1,000 new ones being added every year! Every year America sprays 1.2 billion pounds of pesticides on food crops, dumps 90 billion pounds of toxic waste into waste sites and feeds nine million pounds of antibiotics to the farm animals we eat!

We all come into the world with genetic sensitivities. Everyone has them, but most are not discovered until something triggers a sensitive gene. With the explosion of toxins in our environment since 1900, coupled with the degradation of our diet and lifestyle, it is not surprising that more and more people are reacting to the toxins in our environment. What is surprising is how few people are coming down with environmentally-related cancers.[137] That may be because the cancers are not directly – but indirectly – related to environmental toxins. For example, pesticides, heavy metals, alcohol and other environmental toxins all damage the liver, the main detoxifying organ in your body, and end up

---

[136] Centers for Disease Control, Second National Report on Human Exposure to Environmental Chemicals (31 January 2003).

[137] See Minamoto T, Mai M, Ronai Z. Environmental factors as regulators and effectors of multistep carcinogenesis. Carcinogenesis 1999;20(4):519-27; Cummings JH, Bingham SA. Diet and the prevention of cancer. BMJ 1998;317:1636-40.

compromising your immune system. As a result, you are more vulnerable to cancer.

If you grew up on a farm which uses pesticides, you, your siblings and your parents have a 200 to 400 percent increased risk of developing breast cancer. We all think of farms as bucolic and clean, healthy places to live, but due to the heavy use of chemicals on crops, farming can be deadly.

In the 1970s, there was a study conducted in which animals were fed two percent of their diet from red dye, sodium cyclamate or an emulsifier. The animals that were fed just one additive showed no harmful effects at all. The animals that were fed two of the additives showed balding fur, diarrhea and retarded weight gain. The animals that were fed all three additives were dead within two weeks.[138] Parenthetically, these individual additives were all FDA approved at the time.

In a similar fashion, it was recently reported that Parkinson's disease has been linked to the exposure of not one, but a combination of pesticides, namely paraquat and organophosphate.[139]

What this illustrates is that toxins, when taken together, amplify their toxicity in a synergistic fashion in ways we do not understand and cannot account for.

Of course, we are well-equipped to deal with even heavy loads of multiple toxins in the environment and that is where diet and lifestyle come in because both can speed the exit of toxins from your body and keep your toxic load so low that you will never develop cancer as a result of environmental influences – directly or indirectly. But if you have a lousy diet and lifestyle, the toxins will remain in your body, your toxic load will become heavier and your immune system will become increasingly compromised. This circular, cumulative pattern can result in cancer.

How do we know this is true? Because we know that certain groups who live in highly polluted areas, but follow good diets and lifestyles, have extremely low rates of cancer[140] compared to the general population.

It has long been reported that women who live in breast cancer "hot spots" were at increased risk of breast cancer because they lived near hazardous chemical sites or powerful electrical plants. It turns out this isn't the case at all. Women in those areas with higher risk were wealthy and had higher estrogen levels – directly the result of their affluent, high-fat diets.[141]

The bottom line? If you can reverse cancer with diet and lifestyle changes, then isn't diet and lifestyle the main cause of cancer? Of course it is! Sure, pollution can cause cancer, but we get thousands of cancer cells in our body every day as a result of our interaction with the environment. The more important

---

[138] Ershoff, BH, J. of Food Science, vol. 41, p. 949, 1976.

[139] New Study Suggests Chemicals Could Trigger Disease, AP, 11/6/00.

[140] See, for example, C. Rucker and J. Hoffman, The Seventh-Day Adventist Diet; John Robbins, Healthy at 100, Chapter 4 - The Centenarians of Okinawa.

[141] Deborah Winn, Nature Reviews Cancer 5, 986-994 (December 2005).

question is what does our body do with those cancer cells? If it's well-maintained, it will get rid of them with no problem. If it isn't, they will hang around and start multiplying.

Protein

When you ask the typical American, "Where does protein come from?" they'll stammer for a moment and then say something like, "From meat, dairy and eggs." And they'll be dead wrong. Protein doesn't come from any of these sources. All protein on the planet comes from plants. In fact, protein is created by the interaction of sunlight on plants. Although many people don't think plants have protein at all, plants are the mothers of *all* the protein we eat.

Most people think only animal products have protein, but the lawn in your front yard is full of protein. You may not recognize it, but a cow would. Herbivores, such as cows, eat plants to get their protein. When carnivores eat herbivores, they are actually eating the protein that originally came from the plants eaten by herbivores. The problem with eating protein from animals is that it comes in a package of saturated fat and cholesterol.

For most Americans, getting enough protein simply means eating animal foods. You'll have doctors and dieticians flatly state that you won't get enough protein by just eating plant foods. Unfortunately, they are following the protein requirements of our government, which have been set by the meat, dairy and egg industries through lobbying efforts. This standard is not only ridiculously high, but also potentially dangerous. But because this standard has the flag wrapped around it, nutritionists and health professionals have taken it as "science" and preach this gospel to the public. In fact, they are mindlessly acting as sales persons for industries selling high-protein foods.

A friend recently went to her nutritionist who said that in order to get the protein her body requires purely from vegetables, she would need to consume more vegetables than she could possibly eat. This is not only scientifically false, but an affront to common sense because if that were true, the human race would not have made it to the modern era. It's extremely easy to meet protein needs on virtually any diet. In fact, you'd have to be starving not to get enough protein eating anything other than a junk food diet.

Here's a simple quiz for you. Which has more protein per calorie? Steak, broccoli or spinach? Spinach has the most protein, then broccoli and steak comes in last place.

The USDA dietary guidelines call for protein levels above 10 percent of total calories. Ten percent is four times what the average adult actually needs (see below). This exaggeration, unfortunately, is not based on human needs, but the needs of food lobbies selling high-protein foods.

The protein in human mother's milk is only five percent of total calories. Mother's milk is providing protein during the fastest growth period humans will ever experience outside the womb. At no other time in our lives will we need a greater amount of protein. In fact, the average adult needs only half that amount, or two and one-half percent of calories from protein.[142] More than five percent protein is not only unnecessary, but also potentially dangerous because it will promote cancer and other degenerative diseases. Just one reason "high protein" diets should be avoided like the plague.

Since 1974, the World Health Organization (WHO) has recognized this, but they doubled their recommendation to 5 percent of total calories in order to account for infants and people who are sick. Guess what? The WHO recommendation is exactly what mother's milk provides.

Now, why would the U.S. Government – or anyone else for that matter – recommend anything greater than five percent? Unfortunately, any protein standard higher than five percent is due to money and lobbying, not science.

Most of us would say, well, there's no harm in getting too much protein. But, in fact, there is potentially great harm because high protein diets can result in kidney disease, osteoporosis, cardiovascular disease and cancers.

If you're eating more protein than your body needs, it's burned as a fuel. Unfortunately, protein is both an inefficient fuel and a dirty fuel. It's inefficient because you have to expend more energy to take protein molecules apart than you do to break down carbohydrates and fats, due to the complicated structure of protein. It's dirty because protein contains nitrogen. Instead of producing clean carbon dioxide and water, burning protein produces nitrogenous residues that not only are irritating to the immune system and toxic to the liver, but also put a big workload on the kidneys. High-protein diets can also cause fatigue, digestive strain and aggravation of allergies and autoimmune diseases.

Given all this, why are our protein requirements so high? There is some dubious "science" behind the political efforts of food industries to raise our protein requirements. This science hinges on studies involving rats. In fact, the USDA protein requirements for Americans are based on the nutritional needs of *rats*. The very first study was done back in 1914, but subsequent studies with rats have continued since then and have formed the basis, i.e., the "science," behind our protein requirements. Obviously, the high-protein food industries embraced these studies as if they were manna from heaven.

In the excitement over these studies, it apparently never occurred to anyone that rats are highly inappropriate for the study of human protein requirements. Rats do not eat like humans, digest food like humans, metabolize food like humans, grow like humans and their protein requirements are not at all like humans. In addition, mother's milk from rats is a whopping 49 percent of calories (vs. five percent for human mother's milk), and the amino acid profiles for rats are not at all like human amino acid profiles. But these incidental facts

---

[142] Minimum protein requirements of adults, Hegsted, D., Am. J. Clin. Nutr. 21: 3520; The amino acid requirements of man. XIII The sparing effect of cystine on methionine requirement, Rose, W.C. and Wixom, R.L., J. Biol. Chem., 216, 763-773.

did not deter the "scientists" from their work and making our protein requirements "rat-like" to this day.

In every study conducted with humans, protein from plant foods exceeded human nutritional requirements. Studies in which humans were fed wheat bread alone – or potatoes alone – or corn alone – or rice alone – have all shown that humans were able to meet their protein needs and get all the essential amino acids they needed.[143] And vegetables have an average protein content of 25 percent of calories, far in excess of what we need.[144] And unlike animal protein, vegetable protein does not cause cancers.[145]

But the rat standard for protein has led us into even more difficulties because people have embraced the notion of a "complete" protein and pointed to eggs as the gold standard. This gold standard, however, is based on the nutritional needs of *rats*. In fact, the human body does quite well on foods containing "incomplete" proteins because the body is smart enough to mix and match amino acids in order to form a complete protein to meet the body's needs. In fact, the first thing the body does when it encounters a "complete" protein is break it apart into an incomplete protein, so it can mix and match amino acids according to current needs. The whole notion of a "complete" protein is outdated, based on worthless "science," and should be discarded because it does not apply to human beings. Nor does the current U.S. government standard for protein.

Soy and Breast Cancer

There has been a lot of controversy over soy and breast cancer. Studies which claim soy increases the risk of breast cancer and encourage tumor growth are based on looking at *refined* soy products and many of these studies are very questionable in the first place.[146] There is no credible evidence linking the whole

---

[143] Kofranyi, E., Jekat, F. and Muller-Wecker, H. (1970). 'The minimum protein requirements of humans, tested with mixtures of whole egg plus potatoes and maize plus beans', Z. Physiol. Chem., 351, 1485-1493; Clark, H.E., Malzer, J.L., Onderka, H.M., Howe, J.M. and Moon, W. (1973). 'Nitrogen balances of adult human subjects fed combinations of wheat, beans, corn, milk, and rice', Am. J. Clin. Nutr., 26, 702-706; Edwards, C.H., Booker, L.K., Rumph, C.H., Wright, W.G. and Ganapathy, S.N. (1971). 'Utilisation of wheat by adult man; nitrogen metabolism, plasma amino acids and lipids', Am. J. Clin. Nutr., 24, 181-193; Lee, C., Howe, J.M., Carlson, K. and Clark, H.E. (1971). 'Nitrogen retention of young men fed rice with or without supplementary chicken', Am. J. Clin. Nutr., 24, 318-323; Kies, C., Williams, E. and Fox, H.M. (1965). 'Determination of first limiting nitrogenous factor in corn protein for nitrogen retention in human adults', J. Nutr., 86, 350-356.
[144] Eat To Live, Joel Fuhrman, M.D., p. 52.
[145] See *Part 3 – No Animal Foods*.
[146] Allred CD, et al. Soy processing influences growth of estrogen-dependent breast cancer tumors. Carcinogenesis. 2004 Sep;25(9):1649-57. For a review of some of the

organic soy bean (endamame) with increased breast (or other) cancer risks. In fact, studies point to decreased cancer risks when consuming whole organic soy beans.[147]

Researchers have theorized that natural soy compounds called isoflavones, which have weak estrogen-like effects, could lower breast cancer risk by binding to estrogen receptors in breast tissue and blocking the cancer-promoting effects of the hormone.

But many experts wonder that with its estrogen-like effects, it may itself promote the growth of estrogen-sensitive cancers (breast and prostate), especially

---

fallacious arguments and agendas of soy-bashers, see www.eatkind.net/wholesoystory.htm.

[147] Messina M, Barnes S: The role of soy products in reducing risk of cancer. J Natl Cancer Inst 1991, 83:541-546; Lee HP, Gourley L, Duffy SW, Esteve J, Lee J, Day NE: Dietary effects on breast-cancer risk in Singapore. Lancet 1991, 337:1197-2000; Barnes S, Grubbs C, Setchell KD, Carlson J: Soybeans inhibit mammary tumors in models of breast cancer; Prog Clin Biol Res 1990, 347::239-253; Messina MJ, Loprinzi CL: Soy for breast cancer survivors: a critical review of the literature. J Nutr 2001, 131:3095S-108S; Jefferson WN, Newbold RR: Potential endocrine-modulating effects of various phytoestrogens in the diet. Nutrition 2000, 16:658-662; An J, Tzagarakis-Foster C, Scharschmidt TC, Lomri N, Leitman DC: Estrogen Receptor beta -Selective Transcriptional Activity and Recruitment of Coregulators by Phytoestrogens. J Biol Chem 2001, 276:17808-17814; Zava DT, Duwe G: Estrogenic and antiproliferative properties of genistein and other flavonoids in human breast cancer cells in vitro. Nutr Cancer 1997, 27:31-40; Wu AH, Yu MC, Tseng CC, Pike MC: Epidemiology of soy exposures and breast cancer risk. Br J Cancer 2008, 98:9-14; Messina M, McCaskill-Stevens W, Lampe JW: Addressing the soy and breast cancer relationship: review, commentary, and workshop proceedings. J Natl Cancer Inst 2006, 98:1275-1284; Yonemoto RH: Breast cancer in Japan and United States: epidemiology, hormone receptors, pathology, and survival. Arch Surg 1980, 115:1056-1062; Morrison AS, Lowe CR, MacMahon B, Ravnihar B, Yuasa S: Some international differences in treatment and survival in breast cancer. Int J Cancer 1976, 18:269-273; Murkies A, Dalais FS, Briganti EM, Burger HG, Healy DL, Wahlqvist ML, Davis SR: Phytoestrogens and breast cancer in postmenopausal women: a case control study. Menopause 2000, 7:289-296; De Lemos M: Safety issues of soy phytoestrogens in breast cancer patients. J Clin Oncol 2002, 20:3040-1; Murphy PA, Song T, Buseman G, Barua K, Beecher GR, Trainer D, Holden J: Isoflavones in retail and institutional soy foods. J Agric Food Chem 1999, 47:2697-2704; Boker LK, Van der Schouw YT, De Kleijn MJ, Jacques PF, Grobbee DE, Peeters PH: Intake of dietary phytoestrogens by Dutch women. J Nutr 2002, 132:1319-1328; Takashima N, Miyanaga N, Komiya K, More M, Akaza H: Blood isoflavone levels during intake of a controlled hospital diet. J Nutr Sci Vitaminol (Tokyo) 2004, 50:246-252; Brzezinski A, Adlercreutz H, Shaoul R, Rösler R, Shmueli A, Tanos V, Schenker JG: Short-term effect of phytoestrogen-rich diet on postmenopausal women. Menopause 1997, 4:89-94.

for those people who already have cancer.[148] While soy isoflavones do function as weak estrogens in animal and test tube studies, most of these experiments use unrealistically large amounts of isoflavones – equivalent to *five to sixteen times the amount commonly consumed in Asia. And this is the basic problem with studies linking soy with breast cancer.*

In fact, studies point to decreased cancer risks when consuming whole soy beans.[149] One recent study showed a 13 percent drop in PSA after just one month of adding two ounces of soy each day to the diet.[150] Two ounces a day, by the way, is the typical amount of soy eaten in traditional Chinese and Japanese diets.[151] Breast and prostate cancer rates are four to six times lower in Japan and China than in Western countries, and laboratory studies have shown that isoflavone from soy can inhibit the growth of both breast and prostate cancer tissues.[152]

A recent analysis has concluded that soy isoflavones' estrogen-like effects are probably too weak to have any significant consequence on breast tissue in healthy women, even breast cancer survivors.[153] As the authors stated, "Overall, there is little clinical evidence to suggest that isoflavones will increase breast cancer risk in healthy women or worsen the prognosis of breast cancer patients."

Given all the controversy, however, you may not be at ease with soy, even the whole, organic bean eaten in moderate amounts. There is a very easy solution to this dilemma: Completely eliminate it from your diet. It's as simple as that because there are many other foods to choose from on a plant-based diet that will give you what you need, without having to consume soy. You can also try our soy substitute. See *Part 4 – Soy Sauce Substitute.*

Problems with the Glycemic Index

One of the latest trends in nutrition is a simple-minded, single-variable analysis called the Glycemic Index (GI), which almost every major authority in the country has embraced – including those recommending diets for cancer

---

[148] Newbold R. Uterine adenocarcinoma in mice treated neonatally with genistein. Cancer Res. 2001 Jun 1;61(11):4325-8; Cassileth BR, Vickers AJ. Soy: an anticancer agent in wide use despite some troubling data. Cancer Invest. 2003;21(5):817-8.

[149] Messina MJ, Barnes S. The role of soy products in reducing risk of cancer. J Natl Cancer Inst 1991;83:541-6.

[150] See Dalias, F. Urology, September 2004; vol 64, pp 510-515; Kumar, N. Prostate, May 2004; vol 59; pp 141-147.

[151] Nagata C, Takatsuka N, Kurisu Y, Shimizu H. Decreased serum total cholesterol concentration is associated with high intake of soy products in Japanese men and women. J Nutr. 1998 Feb;128(2):209-13.

[152] Adlercreutz H. Phyto-oestrogens and cancer. Lancet Oncol. 2002 Jun;3(6):364-73.

[153] Mark J Messina, Charles E Wood. Soy isoflavones, estrogen therapy, and breast cancer risk: analysis and commentary. Nutrition Journal 2008, 7:17 (3 June 2008).

patients – despite its serious flaws. Why have they embraced such a flawed tool? Because it has the air of "science" behind it – the GI categorizes foods by simple numbers. Hence, a food can be categorized by a number and placed on a scale. Unfortunately, the GI is of little practical value, despite the fact that there are a number of diets out there based solely on this dubious tool.

The Glycemic Index was designed to measure the effect of a *single food* on blood sugar levels. And that is a big problem. If we were to eat a single food for a meal, the GI might be of limited value. Unfortunately, I've never even heard of anyone who eats a single food for a meal. Factors which throw off the GI in the real world are the mix of fiber, fat and protein in the foods comprising a meal, how refined the ingredients are, whether the food was cooked, fried, how ripe a fruit is, etc.

Another problem is that the GI may predict the effect of a single food on blood sugar levels, but it does not accurately predict how much insulin the body will release in response to a rise in blood sugar. And high insulin levels are associated with increased cancer risks,[154] as well as diabetes and other diseases. Because of this, the GI produces very strange results. Lentils, which are good according to the index, actually provoke *higher insulin levels* than white potatoes, which are bad, according to the index. A fried potato, containing artery-clogging trans-fats, is better than a baked potato. Adding vinegar to a meal can lower the GI of any food and – believe it or not – adding sugar to a food has *no effect* on the index. Ice cream, according to the index, is better for you than whole wheat bread. Sugar-sweetened chocolate is better for you than carrots and a Mars candy bar is better for you than a potato.

Advocates of high-protein diets say that eating carbohydrates raises insulin levels and therefore causes weight gain, while eating animal proteins and fats does not. They are dead wrong. Beef raises insulin levels more than *refined,* white pasta and *27 times* more than brown rice. And fish raises insulin levels more than whole grain bread.[155]

In fact, most of the foods with low GI's are fruits, vegetables, beans and whole grains, the very foods such high-fat (low-carb) diets say you should avoid.

This is just a small sampling of the incoherent contradictions involved with the Glycemic Index that not only defy common sense, but science. The GI is so unreliable that the American Diabetes Association does not recommend using the index in the prevention or treatment of diabetes. Because of all these contradictions, the GI is of little practical value in determining what you should

---

[154] For example, Deborah Josefson. High insulin levels linked to deaths from breast cancer. BMJ 2000;320:1496; Boyd DB. Insulin and cancer. Integr Cancer Ther. 2003 Dec;2(4):315-29; Gunter MJ, et al. Insulin, Insulin-Like Growth Factor-I, and Risk of Breast Cancer in Postmenopausal Women. Journal of the National Cancer Institute 2008 [Epub 30 Dec].
[155] Fad Diets Versus Dietary Guidelines. American Institute for Cancer Research. 02/11/02:12.

be eating and boils down to little more than a red herring that proponents of high-protein diets are using to distract people from good nutrition.

There is a better, simpler and more reliable measure. Instead of focusing on numbers, choose whole, natural plant foods and you will always be eating the best foods you can buy.

Calcium Needs, Osteoporosis and Acidic Diets

"In fact, the scientific literature states clearly that a 'calcium deficiency disease' due to a low calcium intake from natural diets simply does not exist. In other words, all diets provide adequate calcium to meet our health needs...."
– John A. McDougall, M.D.

Many people, particularly women, think they will not get enough calcium if they eliminate dairy products from their diet. This is the result of brain-washing by the dairy industry, so we need to address this.

Your entire body chemistry changes according to the type of food you eat and that has consequences to your health. Because of our change in diet during the last century, American bodies have become very acidic and virtually all degenerative diseases ranging from cancers to tooth decay are associated with excess acidity in our bodies.

Blood acid levels are measured on a pH scale from 1 to 14. Ideally, your blood should be slightly alkaline at 7.4. A soda, for example, has a pH of 2 and is highly acidic, whereas tap water has a pH of 8.4 and is very alkaline.

There are three ways to make your blood less acidic: First, eat more plant foods because plant foods are alkaline and have a higher percentage of water than other foods. Second, drink more water. Not water containing anything else, just plain, simple water. Third, eliminate foods from your diet that make the blood acidic.

The major acid-forming foods in our diets include animal proteins,[156] soft drinks, sugar, salt, caffeine and alcohol. Americans consume too much of all these products. In the case of sodium, we get most of it not from table salt, but indirectly in packaged and processed foods. In fact, dairy products and processed meat are the biggest sources of sodium in the American diet.

---

[156] Advocates of high-protein diets will claim that animal protein has no effect on bone loss. To support this claim, they will quote the work of Herta Spencer, who published two oft-quoted studies, which were badly flawed and biased studies. The root of the flaws and bias? One was paid for by the National Dairy Council (Spencer H. Effect of a high protein (meat) intake on calcium metabolism in man. Am J Clin Nutr. 1978 Dec;31(12):2167-80) and the other by the National Livestock and Meat Board (Spencer H. Further studies of the effect of a high protein diet as meat on calcium metabolism. Am J Clin Nutr. 1983 Jun;37(6):924-9).

High acidity is bad for a number of reasons. First, high acid levels make our bodies more cancer friendly by reducing the delivery of oxygen to cells. In addition, cancer cells love highly acidic environments and do not do well in healthy, alkaline environments. Second, a highly acidic environment disrupts the function of enzymes and the digestion of food. Undigested food gets passed into the colon and sits there, rotting, and this can lead to toxic buildups and a number of health problems. Third, when blood becomes too acidic, our bodies pull calcium from our bones and teeth to neutralize the acid and this contributes to bone loss, or osteoporosis. The body also pulls water from cells to neutralize high acid levels and this leads to cell dehydration, which many experts believe is the number one cause of premature aging.

The way Americans consume antacids is a reflection of just how acidic our diet has become; but taking a calcium pill to neutralize high acid levels is treating a symptom. If you want to eliminate the problem, you'll have to radically cut back on acidic foods.

By continually eating foods which cause high blood acid levels, we put our bodies in a state of constantly having to neutralize this acid by using the calcium stored up in our bones. Animal proteins are one of the most acid-forming foods in existence and because of our high-protein diets, the biggest cause of high-acid levels. One reason dairy products are poor choices for calcium is because they contain excessively high amounts of protein. Cow's milk has over three times more protein than human mother's milk. It was, after all, designed for a calf that will weigh over 300 pounds within a year of its birth.

When you consume dairy products, the calcium simply passes through your body and ends up in the toilet – and your blood is even more acidic because of the protein. Low-fat dairy products are highest in protein, so you may lower your fat intake, but you will raise your blood acid level and this will contribute to bone loss. Skim milk, for example, contains almost twice the amount of protein as whole milk. And because of the high sodium content of dairy products, they provide a double-boost to your acid levels.

In short, consuming dairy products turns out to be the worst possible way to build strong bones. You don't need the sodium, the fat, the acidic proteins, the cholesterol – and you don't need the excess calcium, which can result in painful kidney stones.

The cause of osteoporosis is *not* a lack of calcium in the diet, regardless of the advertising from the dairy industry. Populations that consume the highest amount of calcium have the highest rates of osteoporosis. In fact, the more calcium they consume, the higher their rates of osteoporosis. Conversely, the countries with the *least* amount of calcium consumption have the lowest rates of osteoporosis. Obviously, something else is going on because it's not a lack of calcium that's causing osteoporosis.

What gives? Although Americans are swimming in calcium, the World Health Organization has yet to document a single case of calcium deficiency anywhere in the world.[157] In fact, there has not been a single recorded case of calcium deficiency of a dietary origin in the history of the entire planet.[158] Yet, the dairy industry tells Americans they have a calcium deficiency.

The problem, of course, is that the dairy industry has set U.S. standards for calcium consumption sky high through lobbying efforts. The calcium scare that has been going on in this country is, without question, one of the biggest nutritional scams ever conceived. If you think this is an outrageous statement, then show me a single case of calcium deficiency of a dietary origin. (If you're thinking of rickets, that disease is caused by a lack of vitamin D, not a lack of calcium.)

You'll hear health authorities say that women should get between 1,000 and 1,500 mg of calcium per day, while men should get 1,000 mg per day. What would these health authorities say to men and women throughout the world who get only 200 mg a day and have bones much stronger than Americans? In fact, 70-year-old women in Third World countries who have nursed multiple children have bones stronger than most 40-year-old women in this country. And they get their calcium from plant foods, not dairy products.

Osteoporosis is *not* genetic and you don't have to suffer bone loss if you change your exercise and eating habits. When people say it runs in the family, it simply means the family has led a sedentary lifestyle over generations. Many women, including Dr. Ruth Heidrich (interviewed in the film *Eating*), increased their bone mass during and after menopause without dairy products or hormone replacement therapy.

Bones are just like muscles. The single best thing you can do to prevent (and reverse) osteoporosis is to start exercising your bones, because *a lack of physical activity is the primary cause of osteoporosis.*

Acidic diets will cause bone loss, but not as rapidly as a lack of exercise. People who argue that acidic diets are the primary cause of bone loss have a big flaw in their argument: There are lots of meat-eaters with strong bones. This is because their activity levels strengthen their bones, despite a bad diet. Also, obese women and men never get osteoporosis because they get lots of weight-bearing exercise just carrying their bodies around, regardless of their diet and calcium intake. Lighter women and men have increased chances of osteoporosis simply because their bodies don't have enough weight – unless they run or jog to add stress to their bones. In other words, lighter men and women need to engage in weight-bearing activity in order to strengthen their bones. Swimming is a good

---

[157] The Pritikin Program for Diet & Exercise, Nathan Pritikin, M.D., p. 44.

[158] McDougall's Medicine, John A. McDougall, M.D., p. 70; The McDougall Program, John A. McDougall, M.D., p. 48, Calcium Requirements in man: a critical review, C. Paterson, Postgrad Med J. 54:244, 1978; The human requirement of calcium: should low intakes be supplemented? A. Walker, Am J. Clin Nutr, 25:518, 1972; Symposium on human calcium requirements: Council on Foods and Nutrition, JAMA 185:588, 1963; Modern Nutrition in Health and Disease, 5th ed, Goodhart and Shils, 1973, p. 274.

illustration of how a lack of stress on bones plays out – because runners have higher femur bone densities than swimmers.

It's never been proven that a plant-based diet alone can reverse osteoporosis. It has been proven that exercise reverses osteoporosis. In fact, NASA regularly reverses osteoporosis in astronauts when they return to earth – with an exercise program, not a change in diet. In fact, on that basis alone, exercise is the most proven way to reverse bone loss. (Osteoporosis is a potentially huge problem for long-term space flight because, due to the lack of gravity, NASA is afraid they'd end up with boneless astronauts!)

There are no studies, that I am aware of, which factor both exercise and diet into the equation to determine which is most important. There are, however, hundreds – if not thousands – of studies which show far more dramatic differences in bone density between those who get regular exercise and those who do not.[159] And those differences are gigantic compared to studies that show differences in bone density between people eating different diets. On that basis alone, one has to conclude that exercise is the most important factor affecting bone density. The effect of weight-bearing activity on bone density are extraordinarily well-documented and have consistently shown the same results over decades, regardless of diet.

A recent study showed that varying levels of calcium intake, ranging from 500 mg a day to 1800 mg a day, had *absolutely no effect on bone strength*. It was the *exercise* women got that was the key determinant in building strong bones.[160]

We're worrying about vitamin A and vitamin D and getting enough calcium – all these worries – but no one is worrying about getting enough exercise. Our worries are solely the result of advertising by the dairy industry and the government, which sponsors the dairy industry. To think you can just eat your way out of osteoporosis or take calcium supplements is ridiculous.

Don't worry about calcium. Do worry about exercise. We have this crazy idea that somehow cows produce calcium. They're simply storage systems for the calcium they get from the plants they eat. Calcium comes from the earth – like other minerals – and plant foods are the best place to not only to get calcium, but all the other minerals the body needs. Get your calcium from inexpensive plant foods like the rest of the world does. Plant foods will keep your blood acid level in balance because they're alkaline, not acidic. Like protein, calcium is found in all plant foods and the amounts will easily supply the requirements of growing children and mature adults.

---

[159] JAMA. 2002;288:2300-2306 (41% difference in hip fractures between those women who exercised and those who did not); Aloia, J., Exercise and skeletal health. Journal of American Geriatric Society 29:104, 1981., Smith, E., Physical activity and calcium modalities for bone mineral increase in aged women. Med Sci, Sports Exercise 13:60, 1981, Gymnastics Strengthens Girls' Bones: Study Journal of Pediatrics 2002;141:211-216, Journal of Pediatrics 2002;141:211-216, Smith, E.L., 1982. Exercise for prevention of osteoporosis: A review. The Physician and Sportsmedicine 10(3):72-82.
[160] Study: Exercise Important for Strong Bones, AP, 6/9/04.

Calcium from plant foods is more easily absorbed by bone than calcium from dairy products and unlike dairy, calcium from plants comes in a disease-fighting, low-fat, high-fiber package. Cut back or eliminate all foods that contribute to high-acid levels. Diet and exercise are the keys to preventing and reversing osteoporosis. A change in diet will prevent bone loss and exercise is the *only* way to build strong bones.

To demonstrate just how much calcium is in plant foods, a quick comparison of the calcium content of dairy products versus plant foods is shown below.

Calcium in Milligrams per 100 Calories

Arugula	1,300
Bok choy	1,055
Turnip greens	921
Watercress	800
Collard greens	559
Mustard greens	490
Spinach	450
Broccoli	387
Romaine lettuce	257
Swiss cheese	250
Milk (2-percent)	245
Green onions	240
Okra	213
Cabbage	196
Whole milk	190
Sesame seeds	170
Cheddar cheese	179
American cheese	160
Soybeans	134
Cucumber	108

Surprised to see all those plant foods have more calcium than two percent milk or Swiss cheese? Of course, you're probably saying, "But I would have to eat so much more spinach or kale to get adequate calcium." This is not true because individuals on plant-based diets generally eat as many calories as people eating the standard American diet. In other words, you can get all the calcium you need from the original source of calcium, without getting it second-hand in a package of saturated fat and cholesterol.

Raw and Cooked Foods

There is considerably controversy between "raw foodists" and those who like their foods cooked (or a combination of raw and cooked foods). In *Part 3 - Essential Dietary Guidelines*, I recommend that at least half of your food be uncooked, primarily because fresh, uncooked foods tend to contain more cancer-fighting nutrients than cooked foods.

However, that is not always the case. For example, cooking vegetables increases the content of soluble fiber, which helps fight cancer by decreasing insulin levels, among other things. On the other hand, cooking decreases the content of insoluble fiber, which fights cancer by binding and excreting carcinogens, excess hormones and other toxins.[161] Cooking fights cancer by destroying some of the pesticides present in non-organic produce, but cooking also destroys enzymes that have beneficial effects in digesting foods. Cooking dark green leafy vegetables may destroy half of the antioxidant carotenoids,[162] yet at the same time, cooking may double carotenoid bioavailability.[163]

Raw garlic may be healthier than cooked due to an enzyme called alliinase, which produces a DNA-protecting compound called allicin when chewed in your mouth. When cooked, you absorb little or none of this compound.[164]

An enzyme called myrosinase is produced when chewing raw broccoli. This enzyme can rev up your liver's ability to detoxify carcinogens. Cooking completely deactivates this enzyme, while steaming will produce only a third as much of this enzyme as eating broccoli raw.[165]

Eating cruciferous vegetables (e.g. kale, collards, broccoli, etc.) allows one to absorb two cancer-fighting phytonutrients called isothiocyantes and indoles. With raw cruciferous vegetables, you increase your intake of isothiocyantes, but with cooked, you increase your intake of indoles.

Cruciferous vegetables are the best source of a cancer-fighting nutrient called sulforaphane. In one study, the amount of sulforaphane actually absorbed by human test subjects was ten times higher with raw broccoli than with cooked broccoli.[166]

Raw foodists claim that a raw food diet is healthier, but not for the reasons they provide, which range from eating "live food" or because of the "life force," "living enzymes," "nerve energy," or "chi," in the food. What it boils down to is that foods which can be eaten raw (primarily fruits and vegetables) have

---

[161] Plant Foods in Human Nutrition 55(2000):207.
[162] Journal of the National Cancer Institute 82(1990):282.
[163] Journal of Nutrition 128(1998):913.
[164] Journal of Nutrition 131(2001):1054.
[165] Nutrition and Cancer 38(2000):168.
[166] J Agric Food Chem 2008;56:10505-9.

enormously higher nutrient values, per calorie, than the foods that either have to be, or usually are, cooked. [167] (See *Part 3 - Getting More Bang for the Buck.*)

The bottom line? Eat your greens. At least half of your food should be uncooked and the more the better because of the higher nutrient content, per calorie, of low-fat fruits and vegetables.

---

[167] For an excellent article examining the controversy of raw vs. cooked foods, see William Harris, M.D., www.vegsource.com/harris/raw_vs_cooked.htm.

PART 4 – Meal Preparation

Meal Preparation Rules

One of the beautiful things about the RAVE Diet is its simplicity. There are no complicated formulas or calories to count, so you're eating like a human being, not a target of food advertisers.

Here we present a simple meal preparation formula that will provide you with filling meals, made with a wide variety of nutritious foods, that will keep you happy, healthy and feeling full.

The RAVE Diet food pyramid, shown below, depicts the types of foods you can eat and the general proportions.

The RAVE Diet Food Pyramid

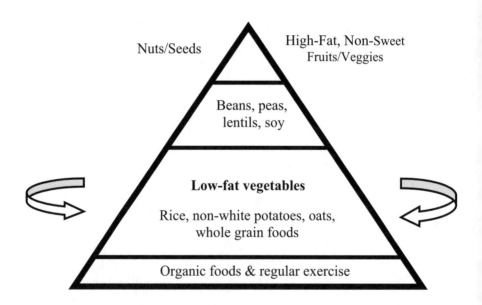

At the top of the pyramid are foods with a high fat to fiber ratio. As you move down the pyramid, the amount of fat generally decreases, relative to the amount of fiber and micronutrients. The fat to fiber ratio increases as you go up the pyramid, which accounts for the declining proportions. The amount of micronutrients per calorie also declines as you go up the pyramid.

At the very top are foods such as nuts and seeds, followed by high-fat non-sweet fruits, such as avocados and olives. Great foods, but about 80 percent fat, so go easy on them.

The higher protein foods tend to be beans, peas, lentils and soy. (See *Part 3 – Soy and Breast Cancer* for more on soy.) These are near the top of the pyramid because they are still high in fat content, so you need to watch the proportions. And you don't need to eat these foods to get protein. Protein is found in *all* foods and you'll get more than adequate amounts – as well as all other essential nutrients – by just eating any variety of these foods.

Next are low-fat vegetables, which is the most important food group for fighting cancer and keeping you looking and feeling young. *Your diet should center on **low-fat vegetables**, particularly green vegetables.*

Next are rice, non-white potatoes and whole grain foods. Use these as meat substitutes to fill you up. Always choose brown rice (or another *whole* grain rice), never eat white rice – or any other food that's white for that matter – and always eat potatoes with the skin. Sweet potatoes are only 11 percent fat, brown rice is 6 percent fat, wild rice is 3 percent fat, barley and bulgur are both 3 percent fat. All of the whole-wheat grains are under 10 percent fat. Compare that with typical (non-fried) servings of rib steak (78% fat), chicken (54% fat), turkey (42% fat) or Atlantic salmon (54% fat), and you can see where we're going with this.

Organic foods and regular exercise are at the base of the pyramid. You must always buy certified organic products because they are much higher in micronutrients. These foods are grown without the use of chemical fertilizers and pesticides. Pesticides, in fact, reduce the amount of antioxidants in plants, so organic foods have higher cancer-fighting nutrients than conventionally grown foods. The reason for this is that plants use their antioxidants in an effort to defend themselves against pesticides, thus lowering the antioxidants available to consumers.[1] (For more on organic foods, see *Part 4 – Reading Labels & Ingredients.*)

Spices, herbs and sauces are throughout the pyramid. Use these to give your food added flavor. Spices and herbs, in particular, are rich in cancer-fighting nutrients and can turn plain-tasting foods into fabulous tasting foods. (See Part 4 – *Flavorings.*) If you're not familiar with spices, you can start with Italian Seasoning, as that is universally liked, and branch out from there. If you think eating a plant-based diet is boring, you'll be pleasantly surprised once you learn how to use herbs and spices.

It's a lot easier than you think to follow the RAVE Diet. All you have to do is choose your favorite foods from the pyramid, follow the proportions – and Bingo! – you're doin' the *RAVE*. It's really as simple as that. Remember, plant foods are medicines. The more you eat, the healthier you're going to be. And if

---

[1] American Chemical Society Press Release, 3/3/03, printed in Journal of Agricultural and Food Chemistry, 2/26/03.

you ever get stumped about what to eat, see *Food Lists*, which shows a sampling of just how many foods are available with the RAVE Diet.

Some people like to have meal plans, i.e., what to eat for the next two weeks, for example. I personally don't like them because what do you do after two weeks? If you want a meal plan, it's very simple to put together. Just select a recipe for breakfast, lunch and dinner for the next two weeks. You can select them at random, in sequence, or repeat the same ones. It's that easy.

Here are a few simple examples of the pyramid:

Breakfast
    Condiments
    Nuts
    Juice/smoothie
    Oatmeal & breads

Lunch (salad)
    Seasonings/sauces
    Avocado
    Beans
    Low-fat vegetables
    Green leafy salad vegetables

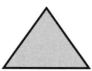

Dinner
    Seasonings/sauces
    Beans/peas
    Low-fat vegetables
    Rice/sweet potatoes/bulgur, etc.

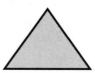

There are an infinite number of variations within the pyramid and, in this sense, there are no rules. You can tailor the diet to meet your specific tastes. The sample recipes contained in this book are just that – samples – because you will discover what you like and how you like to prepare your food on your own. Don't be afraid to substitute recipe ingredients, add vegetables to recipes or change them around. Everyone has their favorite plant foods and you will be able to fit them into the rules very simply. And don't worry about making a mistake. Too much ginger in a recipe, for example, can be easily covered up by adding other spices.

Cooking Without Oil

When sautéing, use about twice as much water (or other oil substitute) as you would oil – and add as necessary. This will vary, depending on what you are sautéing, but with a little experience you will get the hang of it. And remember, you can always add more oil substitute if needed. You'll soon discover you don't need even a drop of oil to make your food delicious – and it won't have that greasy taste, but the nice, natural taste of whole foods.

Cook on low or medium heat to avoid the water (or oil substitute) evaporating too quickly. This will take a little longer than a high-heat oil-based sauté, but it's worth the wait because you're not sending the oil to your hips – or waist – and the food tastes so much cleaner! If you need to brown something, just turn up the heat to high at the end of the cooking, stir the food, and the water will evaporate quickly. Believe it or not, you can make delicious browned home fries using just water. The following are oil substitutes for sautéing and baking:

Oil Substitutes for

> **Sautéing:** water, apple juice, sherry, vegetable stock, wine, vinegars

> **Baking:** any pureed fruit, e.g., applesauce, apple butter, pureed bananas, pureed prunes

With baked goods, use the same amount of substitute, as you would oil. Many use baby food purees as a convenient substitute. Baby food purees work best if the puree is diluted with a little water.

Making Plain Foods Taste Fabulous

To most people, natural whole foods taste rather "plain," at least until your taste buds adjust and you come to enjoy the wide varieties of tastes inherent in whole, natural foods. The easiest and most delicious way to make these foods more exciting is to add seasonings and sauces.

I'm often asked, "How do you liven up your food?" It's easy with seasonings and sauces because there are hundreds you can choose from. What follows is a short list to get you started. The flavors of most whole plant foods are very subtle and they will easily take on whatever seasonings or sauces you care to use. Just be careful with commercial seasonings or custom mixes to make sure there is no added salt in them. You should avoid all salt seasonings, except for salt substitutes, such as Mrs. Dash or Salt Free Spike.

And don't be shy when you're dining out. If you eat a food that tastes delicious, ask the chef what seasonings he used with it.

Here is a short list of some of my favorite commercial seasonings:

Coriander	Italian Seasoning
Cumin	Mint
Curry	Mustard
Fajita Seasoning	Oregano Leaf
Hungarian Hot Paprika	

Flavorings

The following lists various foods and the seasonings that are typically used with them. We then give a short list of seasonings, sauces, salad dressings, condiments and sweeteners. Of course, if you have a favorite seasoning, it can go with practically anything – because it's *your* favorite.

Seasonings

Beans
Avocado, cayenne, chili, cumin, epazote, Mexican oregano, parsley, pepper, savory, sage, thyme

Breads
Anise, basil, cardamom, cinnamon, coriander, cumin, dill, garlic, lemon peel, orange peel, poppy, seeds, saffron, thyme, rosemary

Fruits
Anise, black pepper, cardamom, cinnamon, coriander, cumin, ginger, mint

Potatoes, rice
Basil, coriander, dill, oregano, paprika, parsley, poppy seeds, rosemary, thyme

Salads & Dressings
Basil, caraway, celery seed, fennel, garlic, ginger, lemon peel, mint, mustard, oregano, paprika, parsley, rosemary, thyme

Soups
Basil, bay, black pepper, chives, chili, cilantro, cumin, dill, fennel, garlic, paprika, parsley, rosemary, thyme

Sweets
Anise, cardamom, cinnamon, cloves, fennel, ginger, lemon peel, nutmeg, orange peel, rosemary, saffron

Vegetables
Chili, cumin, mustard, curry powder, garam masala, ginger, dill, cilantro, black pepper, garlic, mint, paprika, thyme, turmeric

Here is a description of some of the more common spices and their typical uses.

Allspice: Pungent, spicy, like a mix of nutmeg, cloves and cinnamon. Virtually anything, from salads to desserts.
Anise: Sweet, similar to licorice. Flavoring in cookies, candies and pastries.
Basil: Pungent, somewhat sweet. Tomato dishes, salads, cooked vegetables.
Bay leaves: Bitter, pungent. Soups, stews, tomato sauces. Remove leaf before serving
Black pepper: Pungent, somewhat hot. Virtually anything.
Borage: Mild. Garnish or in salads or in herbal tea mixtures.
Capers: Pungent. In sauces, as a garnish.

Caraway seeds: Sweet, nutty. Cookies and cakes, apple sauce, vinegars.
Cardamom: Sweet, pungent, fragrant, strong taste. Stews, curries.
Cayenne pepper: Very hot. In anything you want to taste hot.
Celery seed: Pungent celery flavor. Flavoring in tomato juice, sauces and soups.
Chervil: Similar to parsley. Flavoring in soups, casseroles, salads.
Chile powder: Spicy, hot. In chili or other spicy dishes.
Chives: Sharp, onion or garlic flavor. Fresh; frozen if fresh not available Garnish, added to salads.
Cilantro: Spicy, sweet or hot. Common ingredient in Mexican salsas.
Cinnamon: Sweet, fragrant. Sweet dishes, curries and stews.
Cloves: Sweet or bittersweet. Sweet dishes or as a contrast in stews and curries.
Coriander: Warm, aromatic. Cakes, cookies, breads, curries.
Cumin: Peppery, aromatic. Soups, stews, sauces.
Curry powder: Hot. Curries.
Dill: Bittersweet, cool. Potatoes, meats, breads, salads, sauces, curries.
Fennel: Similar to anise, but sweeter, lighter, warm. Salads, soups, stews.
Fenugreek: Sweet, somewhat like burnt sugar. Pastries, beverages, syrups.
Garlic: Pungent, onion-like. Roasted, or flavoring for pasta sauces. Good in any dish meal.
Ginger: Mix of pepper and sweetness. Cakes, breads, cookies, Asian dishes.
Green peppercorns: Mild, slightly sweet. Vinegars, in sauces.
Horseradish: Sharp, similar to mustard. As condiment.
Lovage: Similar to celery, but stronger. Use as you would celery, in soups, stews, salads.
Mace: Similar to nutmeg, but stronger. Custards, spice cakes, fruit desserts.
Marjoram: Delicate taste. Soups, stews, marinades.
Mint: Sweet, aromatic, cooling. Salads, vegetables.
Mustard, brown: Sharp, pungent, hotter than yellow mustard. Use as condiment.
Mustard, yellow: Hot, tangy, less of a bite than brown mustard. Use as a condiment.
Nutmeg: Warm, spicy, sweet. Cakes, cookies, sweet potatoes.
Oregano: Delicate taste. Pasta dishes, chili, vegetables, soups.
Paprika: Sweet, warm. Soups, potato salad.
Parsley: Mildly peppery. Garnish in sauces, soups and salads.
Poppy seed: Nutty, aromatic. Muffins, cakes, salad dressings.
Rosemary: Aromatic. Sauces, vegetables.
Saffron: Pungent, aromatic, fragrant. Rice, stews, curries.
Sage: Musty, slightly bitter. Stews, vegetables.
Sesame seed: Nutty. Breads, salad dressings.
Star Anise: Very similar to anise. Flavoring in cookies, candies and pastries.
Summer savory: Cross between thyme and mint, milder than winter savory. Soups, bean dishes.
Tarragon: Sweet, pungent. Vegetables.

Thyme: Minty, lemony. Soups, salads, cooked vegetables.
Turmeric: Pungent, somewhat bitter, warm. Curries. Primary ingredient in yellow commercial mustard.
Vanilla: Sweet, aromatic, fragrant. Desserts.
White pepper: Similar to black peppercorn, milder. As a condiment.
Winter savory: Combination of thyme and mint. Soups, bean dishes, vegetables.

Sauces

You can make your own sauces, of course, but there are hundreds of commercial brands available and more convenient to use. Experiment and mix your favorite sauces together to create a new sauce just for you. Here are just a few of my favorites:

A1 Steak sauce
Barbeque sauce
Black bean sauce
Chipotle sauce
Cranberry sauce
Dijon Mustard
Hoisin sauce
Hot pepper sauce
Plum sauce
Salsa
Tamari (soy sauce - low-sodium, or Bragg Liquid Aminos if sensitive to soy)
Tabasco sauce
Teriyaki sauce (low-sodium)
Tomato sauce
Tomato ketchup
Vegetarian Worcestershire sauce

Note: Ingredients will vary for a particular sauce, depending on who makes it, so inspect the label closely before purchasing.

A Better Tomato Sauce

Most prepared pasta sauces contain oil and are high in sodium. The best way is to simply make your own – and it's incredibly easy.

All you have to do is purchase cans (or jars) of tomato sauce and canned or fresh cut tomatoes. (Note: there should not be oil or sodium added).

Just chop up some of your favorite vegetables (or throw them in a food processor), mix them into the tomato sauce with the tomatoes and add your favorite herbs or just use Italian seasoning and Voila! You have your own pasta sauce.

You can flavor the sauce however you want. I usually add some Tabasco sauce or horseradish to give it a little zing. Or feel free to add any other spices, herbs or sauces for flavor. Once you get it down, you'll have a pasta sauce that tastes the way you like it. I usually just buy the tomato sauce and add whatever I have on hand at the moment. As you'll discover, the taste is much cleaner than the oily stuff sold on the shelf.

If you like it fresher (I do), here is a simple way to make your own tomato sauce from scratch.

Easy Tomato Sauce

6 Roma tomatoes, coarsely chopped
1 clove garlic, minced
1 or 2 sprigs fresh basil leaves
1/4 teaspoon ground black pepper

Combine all the ingredients in the food processor and process to a smooth or chunky sauce as desired.

Condiments

Applesauce	Mustards
Banana chips	Mushrooms
Cilantro	Olives
Corn relishes	Pickles
Ginger	Potatoes
Hummus	Salsa
Lemon juice	Sunflower seeds
Lime juice	Tomato sauce

Salad Dressings Without Oil

Balsamic vinaigrette dressings
Other vinegar-based dressings

Cuisine Perel makes a wide range of vinegar-based dressings that are fabulous. www.gourmetofoldecity.com/perelvinegars.html

Make Your Own[1]

These are quick and simple recipes to make delicious oil-free salad dressings. Simply increase the proportions to make larger amounts. The directions are the same for all dressings: simply combine all ingredients.

Balsamic Vinaigrette

1/3 cup balsamic vinegar
1/4 cup apple cider vinegar
1 tbsp water
2 tsp mustard

Blackstrap-Mustard Vinaigrette

1/4 cup apple-cider vinegar
4-5 tsp blackstrap molasses (unsulfured)
1 tsp mustard

Garlicky-Tomato Dressing

1 garlic clove pressed
1/4 cup vegetable juice
1 tsp lemon juice
1/4 tsp Italian seasoning

Italian Dressing

1/4 cup red-wine vinegar
1 tbsp lemon juice
1/2 tsp dried minced onion
1/4 tsp oregano
1/4 tsp basil
Pinch of thyme
Pinch of garlic powder

---

[1] Some of these recipes were adapted from Mary Clifford, RD , Flavorful Salad Dressings Without the Oil!, Vegetarian Journal May/June 1999 and CancerProject.org.

Mustard-Balsamic Vinaigrette

1/3 cup balsamic vinegar
1/3 cup mustard of choice
1/4 cup apple cider vinegar
1 tsp water

Mustard-Garlic Vinaigrette #1

½ cup rice vinegar
2 tsp mustard
1 garlic clove pressed

Mustard-Garlic Vinaigrette #2
Makes 3-4 cups

2-3 medium garlic cloves
1/2 cup mustard
3 tbsp lemon juice or rice or cider vinegar
3 tbsp water
1 tsp light miso
1 tsp low-sodium Tamari (soy sauce)
1/2 tsp maple syrup
1/2 tsp curry powder

Raspberry Vinaigrette

1 clove garlic
3/4 cup water
1/4 cup raspberry vinegar
1/2 inch sliced shallot
2 tbsp walnuts
1 tsp Dijon mustard
1/4 tsp basil

Tomato Vinaigrette

1 clove garlic pressed
¾ cup tomato juice
3 tbsp apple vinegar
1 tbsp lemon juice
1 tsp mustard

Sweeteners

All of the sweeteners listed below, although healthier than refined sugar, should be used very sparingly, if at all. Ideally, only fresh or dried whole fruits should be used as sweeteners.

Agave nectar
Barley malt syrup
Brown rice syrup
Concentrated fruit juice syrups
Date sugar (ground, dehydrated dates)
Fresh or dried fruits
Maple sugar
Maple syrup
Molasses (black strap-unsulfured)
Organic unrefined cane sugar.
Organic dairy-free chocolate
Sorghum syrup
Turbinado sugar

Soy Sauce Substitute

Molasses
Balsamic vinegar

In a small bowl, mix 2 1/2 parts molasses with 1 part balsamic vinegar. You can vary this to taste.

Bean Preparation

Beans are an excellent source of nutrients. Although they tend to be high in fat, they should be eaten frequently. The most convenient way to eat beans is right from the can, but in the can they are high in sodium and other preservatives, so it is best to avoid that.

Purchasing dry beans in bulk is much healthier (sodium free, preservative free and process free), they are cheaper than canned beans and they are more environmentally friendly (less energy expended in production, less energy expended in recycling and less material used for packaging). And with a little planning, dry beans can be prepped and cooked very easily.

First, always rinse dry beans using a colander and pick out any defective or broken beans or debris, such as twigs, etc.

Next you must soak them. Soaking helps break down the complex sugars (oligosaccharides) in beans, which will greatly reduce or eliminate flatulence. A soaked bean is more likely to retain its maximum nutritional value.

When soaking, beans will rehydrate to at least twice their dry size, so be sure to start with a large enough pot and use about twice the amount of water as beans. How can you tell if a bean is fully soaked? Cut a bean open. If the bean is undersoaked, you'll notice the core is chalky, as if a kernel of rice was in the center. If the bean is fully soaked, it has an even color all the way through.

Quick Soak: Bring a pot of water to boil, add the dry beans and let them boil for about two to three minutes. After boiling, turn off the heat, cover and let them soak in the hot water for one to two hours. After you have soaked them, drain the beans, add fresh water (approx an inch above the beans) and cook until tender.

Long Soak: Put the dry beans in a large bowl or pot of room temperature water (too cold or hot will affect the beans negatively). Add water. Let them sit for 8 to 10 hours, or overnight. After soaking, drain the beans and add fresh water (approx an inch above the beans). Bring to a boil, then reduce the heat and cook until tender. Add seasonings to taste during cook time, if desired.

Cooking times will vary, depending on the bean, but will generally range from 45 minute to an hour and a half. The big exception is soy beans, which can take three to four hours to cook.

Pressure Cooking: When using a pressure cooker, you can either soak the beans or eliminate that step altogether. We recommend soaking because it still helps break down the complex sugars. Either way, put the beans in the pressure cooker, adding three times as much water as beans. Cook at 15 pounds of pressure for 30 minutes for small beans. For large beans, such as limas or fava beans, pressure cook for about 40 minutes. Note: if you have an old pressure cooker, you can eliminate foaming by putting in a strip of kombu (dried seaweed available at health food stores). Newer pressure cookers do not have a problem with foaming.

Fresh Beans:[1] Fresh beans are not as readily available as dry beans, but they can be found in farmer's markets. You will have to first shell the beans before cooking.

There are two basic methods of cooking fresh beans: boiling or steaming. To boil, drop the shelled beans into boiling water and cover. Boil gently for five to ten minutes. To steam, put about an inch of water into the bottom of a saucepan, and then place the beans into a steamer basket (that will fit into the saucepan). Cover the pan and steam over boiling water for five to ten minutes.

Note: after fresh fava beans are cooked, their tough skins are usually peeled and discarded. When left on, they give the beans a bitter flavor. To peel the skins, us a small paring knife and peel away one end. Then squeeze the opposite end and the bean will slip out easily.

Microwaves

Some 90 percent of modern households have microwave ovens and there is a lot of controversy about their safety and what they do to food. You will find countless articles on the internet claiming that microwaving is unsafe. Most of these claims are unsubstantiated. For example, there is the case of Norma Levitt who was given a blood transfusion with blood heated in a microwave oven and died shortly thereafter. People cite this as "proof" the microwave "somehow" altered Ms. Levitt's blood and that was what killed her. In fact, a jury found that Norman Levitt died of a blood clot, not of microwaved blood.[2]

---

[1] This preparation advice is from Zel and Reuben Allen, Vegetarians in Paradise.

[2] www.wyom.state.wy.us/applications/oscn/deliverdocument.asp?citeid=4387 This is the reference to the civil case regarding Norma Levitt. Microwaving blood is never a good idea in the first place. Heating blood with a microwave destroys red blood cells, which can result in "gross hemolysis" of the blood, releasing large amounts of potassium. Excessive potassium, when introduced into the body, can be fatal. This was not the case with Norma Levitt, however.

Surprisingly, there have not been comprehensive studies on the effect of microwave cooking with respect to human health, so we do not have a good basis for judging health concerns in this regard. Despite this and the fact that people have reversed cancers while occasionally microwaving their food, I would recommend you *not* use microwaves at all. In fact, I would recommend you pack your microwave in a box and put it in the garage, so it will not tempt you. Although there is not conclusive evidence that microwaves are unsafe, there is some evidence that they are, so to be on the safe side, I recommend against them. Microwaving is a convenience, not a necessity, so it can easily be discontinued.

In one very small study,[3] it was found that microwaved food produced changes in the subjects' blood and immune function. These included a decrease in hemoglobin, an increase in hemotocrit and leukocytes and a decrease in lymphocytes. There was also an increase in the activity of certain bacteria in the food as well as the appearance of altered cells resembling the pathogenic stages that occur in the early development of some cancers. In the food itself, there was increased acidity, damaged protein molecules, enlarged fat cells and decreased amounts of folic acid.

Collecting, freezing and reheating breast milk is standard practice in most neonatal units in the US. In a study by Stanford University School of Medicine, it was found that human breast milk loses some of its abilities to fight infection when reheated with a microwave oven. It also weakened antibodies and proteins that inhibit bacterial growth and help infants ward off infection.[4]

Chemicals used in "microwave safe" packaging, such as found in microwave popcorn, pizza, etc. can migrate into food.[5] The FDA has been made aware of this, but they have failed to regulate the problem.

There are also claims that nutrients are lost when microwaving food. This is not supported by scientific evidence. The reality is that *every* cooking method can destroy vitamins and other nutrients in food. The factors that determine the extent of destruction are how long the food is cooked, how much liquid is used and the cooking temperature, not whether the food was microwaved.

For example, a recent study[6] showed that microwaving broccoli removed anywhere from 74 to 97 percent of flavonoids, a vital nutrient that fights not just

---

[3] Bernard H. Blanc and Hans U. Hertel, "Influence on Man: Comparative Study About Food Prepared Conventionally and in the Microwave Oven," Raum & Zeit, 3(2): 1992.

[4] Quan R, et al., Effects of microwave radiation on anti-infective factors in human milk, Pediatrics. 1992 Apr;89(4 Pt 1):667-9; Microwaving Breast Milk, Microwave News, May/June 1992, p. 14. See also, G. Lubec et al., Aminoacid Isomerisation and Microwave Exposure, Lancet 2(8676):1392-93, 1989.

[5] David Steinman and Samuel S. Epstein, M.D., Safe Shopper's Bible (New York: Macmillan, 1995).

[6] F Vallejo, FA Tomás-Barberán, C García-Viguera, Phenolic compound contents in edible parts of broccoli inflorescences after domestic cooking, Journal of the Science of Food and Agriculture, Volume 83 Issue 14 , Pages 1389 - 1538 (November 2003). See

cancer, but cardiovascular and other diseases. However, the nutrients were not "lost," but were simply leached out of the vegetable and into the water that was used for cooking. If you include the water with your meal, you have theoretically not lost any nutrients at all. In comparison, boiling broccoli removed 66 percent of the flavonoids and pressure cooking leached out 47 percent. Quick and simple steaming was the best method and had only minimal losses. The loss of micronutrients by any cooking method is one reason I recommend at least half of your food be eaten uncooked. (See *Part 3 – Essential Dietary Guidelines.*)

Environmental Exposure to Microwaves

While many are concerned about microwaving their food, they are also busy talking on their cell phones, computing over WiFi (wireless) connections and exposing themselves to microwaves in the environment. The ambient radiation level has increased dramatically over the last few decades and this can potentially be more dangerous than microwaving food.

Symptoms known to be caused by exposure to electromagnetic radiation – depending on frequency, duration, and exposure levels – range from decreased stamina, memory problems, fatigue, sleep disturbances, headaches, eye sensitivities, increased allergies and dizziness to insomnia, swollen lymph nodes, depression, loss of appetite, hypoxia (lack of oxygen getting to the tissues), vision problems, weakened immune system, frequent urination, night sweats and so on.[7] Not surprisingly, such symptoms often appear suddenly in people who have had a cell phone tower installed near their home.

---

also, Fumio Watanabe, et al., Effects of Microwave Heating on the Loss of Vitamin B12 in Foods, J. Agric. Food Chem., 1998, 46 (1), pp 206–210.

[7] Becker, R.O., The Body Electric, pp. pp. 314-315; Cherry N. (1996). "Swiss shortwave transmitter study sounds warning." Electromagnetics Forum , Vol. 1, No. 2 Article 10; Microwave News. Sept/Oct. page 14; Kolodynski AA, Kolodynska VV. (1996). "Motor and psychological functions of school children living in the area of the Skrunda Radio Location Station in Latvia." Sci Total Environ. Feb 2;180(1):87-93; Santini R, Santini P, Danze JM, Le Ruz P, Seigne M. (2002). "Investigation on the health of people living near mobile telephone relay stations: I/Incidence according to distance and sex." Pathol Biol (Paris). [Article in French] Jul; 50(6):369-73; Al-Khlaiwi T, Meo SA. (2004). "Association of mobile phone radiation with fatigue, headache, dizziness, tension and sleep disturbance in Saudi population." Saudi Medical Journal, Jun; 25(6): 732-6; Bortkiewicz A, Zmyslony M, Szyjkowska A, Gadzicka E. (2004). "Subjective symptoms reported by people living in the vicinity of cellular phone." Med Pr.; 55 (4):345-51. See also Do You Have Microwave/EMR Sickness? by Paul Raymond Doyon. Much of this discussion and references is based on this article. It can be found on the internet by searching the title.

160 – Healing Cancer From Inside Out

Studies on the effects of ambient radiation in microwave ovens, cell phones, cordless phones, fluorescent lighting, transformers, cell phone towers, electrical substations and power lines have shown that exposure can induce the following:

- An abnormal flux of calcium into and out of cells, which can trigger or aggravate allergic reactions.[8]
- An increase in allergies[9] due to an increase in the production of histamine, the chemical responsible for allergic reactions.[10]
- An increase in immunoglobulin antibodies in the body, which are responsible for triggering an allergic reaction to a particular substance or protein.[11]
- Mitochondria dysfunction, which is the powerhouse of human cells. This may cause fatigue as well as other problems.[12]

---

[8] Amara S, Abdelmelek H & Sakly M. (2004). "Effects of acute exposure to magnetic field ionic composition of frog sciatic nerve." Pakistani Journal of Medical Science. 20(2) 91-96; Cellphones - a boon to modern society or a threat to human health? An interview with Dr Neil Cherry, NZine (online), 6/01/03.

[9] Kimata H. (2003). Enhancement of allergic skin wheal responses in patients with atopic eczema/dermatitis syndrome by playing video games or by a frequently ringing mobile phone. Eur J Clin Invest. Jun: 33(6):513-7; Kimata H. (2005). Microwave radiation from cellular phones increases allergen-specific IgE production. Allergy. Jun;60(6):838-9; Kimata H. (2002). Enhancement of allergic skin wheal responses by microwave radiation from mobile phones in patients with atopic eczema/dermatitis syndrome. Int Arch Allergy Immunol. Dec;129(4):348-50.

[10] Johansson O, et al., Cutaneous mast cells are altered in normal healthy volunteers sitting in front of ordinary TVs/PCs--results from open-field provocation experiments. J Cutan Pathol. 2001 Nov;28(10):513-9; Johansson O, Hilliges M, Han SW. A screening of skin changes, with special emphasis on neurochemical marker antibody evaluation, in patients claiming to suffer from screen dermatitis as compared to normal healthy controls. Exp Dermatol (1996) 5: 279-285.

[11] Bergier L, Lisiewicz J, et al. Effect of electromagnetic radiation on T-lymphocyte subpopulations and immunoglobulin level in human blood serum after occupational exposure. Med Pr.;41(4):211-5 (1990); Dmoch A., Moszczynski P. (1998). Levels of immunoglobulin and subpopulations of T lymphocytes and NK cells in men occupationally exposed to microwave radiation in frequencies of 6-12 GHz. Med Pr. 49(1):45-9; Moszczynski P, Lisiewicz J, Dmoch A, Zabinski Z, Bergier L, Rucinska M, Sasiadek U. The effect of various occupational exposures to microwave radiation on the concentrations of immunoglobulins and T lymphocyte subsets. Wiad Lek. 52(1-2):30-4 (1999); Yuan ZQ, et al. Effect of low intensity and very high frequency electromagnetic radiation on occupationally exposed personnel. Zhonghua Lao Dong Wei Sheng Zhi Ye Bing Za Zhi. Aug: 22(4):267-9 (2004); Kimata H. Microwave radiation from cellular phones increases allergen-specific IgE production. Allergy. Jun;60(6):838-9 (2005).

[12] Gerald Goldberg, M.D., Would You Put Your Head in a Microwave Oven?, 2006; Buchachenko AL, et al. New mechanisms of biological effects of electromagnetic fields. Biofizika, May-Jun;51(3):545-52 (2006).

- A decrease in the numbers of Natural Killer (NK) cells, the body's first line of defense against pathogens and extremely important when fighting cancer.[13]
- A weakened immune system.[14]
- An increase in viruses, bacteria, mold, parasites, and yeast in the blood of the human host.
- "Subliminal" stress (since the body does not know it is under stress), which causes the adrenal glands to excrete abnormally greater amounts of cortisol and adrenaline. This can lead to irritability and hyperactivity. If continued it could eventually lead to adrenal exhaustion, which is commonly found in chronic fatigue syndrome.[15]
- A decrease in levels of the brain hormone norepinephrine,[16] which is essential for control of the autonomic nervous system. If not working properly, the body will have trouble regulating its temperature.[17] People with chronic fatigue syndrome have been found to have a disturbed circadian core body temperature.[18] A decrease in norepinephrine levels has also been connected to short-term memory disturbances, ADHD and depression.
- Alters the production of the brain hormone melatonin, which is necessary for proper sleep.[19]
- Changes the level of the brain hormone, dopamine (or dopamine transporters), which has been linked with depression and restless leg syndrom.[20]

---

[13] Smialowicz RJ, Rogers RR, Garner RJ, Riddle MM, Luebke RW, Rowe DG. Microwaves (2,450 MHz) suppress murine natural killer cellactivity. Bioelectromagnetics. 4(4):371-81 (1983); Nakamura H, et al. Effects of exposure to microwaves on cellular immunity and placental steroids in pregnant rats. Occup Environ Med, Sep;54(9):676-80 (1997); Yang H.K., et al. Effects of microwave exposure on the hamster immune system. I. Natural killer cell activity. Bioelectromagnetics. 1983; 4(2): 123-39.

[14] Levitt, B. Blake, Electromagnetic Fields, pp. 128-129, 1995. See also, Immune system attacked by mobile phones, BBC News, October 15, 1998.

[15] Levitt BB. Electromagnetic Fields, 1995.

[16] Takahashi A, et al. Aspects of hypothalamic neuronal systems in VMH lesion-induced obese rats." Journal of Autonomic Nervous System. Aug;48(3):213-9 (1994).

[17] Gandhi VC, Ross DH. Alterations in alpha-adrenergic and muscarinic cholinergic receptor binding in rat brain following nonionizing radiation." Radiation Res. Jan; 109(1):90-9 (1987).

[18] Tomoda A, et al. Disturbed circadian core body temperature rhythm and sleep disturbance in school refusal children and adolescents." Biol Psychiatry. Apr 1; 41(7): 810-3 (1997).

[19] Altpeter E.S, et al. Effect of short-wave (6-22 MHz) magnetic fields on sleep quality and melatonin cycle in humans: the Schwarzenburg shut-down study. Bioelectromagnetics. Feb: 27(2):142-50 (2006).

- An abnormal drop in the levels of the neurotransmitter acetylcholine, which has been linked to a number of neurological and neuromuscular disorders.[21]
- Alters regional cerebral blood flow, which corresponds to altered blood flow in conditions such as chronic fatigue syndrome.[22]

In addition to the above, recent studies have found links between cell phone use and the development of brain tumors and other cancers.[23] One of these studies found that your risk of developing a brain tumor is 240 percent higher if you spend an hour a day on your cell over several years, versus someone who never used one.

Of course, all these studies show "links" and not conclusive proof or causation. Conversely, there have also been studies[24] in which mammary-tumor-prone animals were subjected to chronic, long-term exposure of microwave bandwidths and there were no differences between the exposed animals and the control animals. Other studies[25] have exposed animal fetus' to microwave radiation to see if it affected their brain development and it did not.

---

[20] Brown AS, Gershon S. Dopamine and depression. J Neural Transm Gen . Sect. 91(2-3): 75-109 (1993); Allen R. Dopamine and iron in the pathophysiology of restless legs syndrome (RLS). Sleep Medicine, Jul;5(4):385-91 (2004).

[21] Omura Y, Losco M. Electro-magnetic fields in the home environment (color TV, computer monitor, microwave oven, cellular phone, etc) as potential contributing factors for the induction of oncogen C-fos Ab1, oncogen C-fos Ab2, integrin alpha 5 beta 1 and development of cancer, as well as effects of microwave on amino acid composition of food and living human brain." Acupunct Electrother Res. Jan-Mar;18(1):33-73 (1993); Testylier G, et al. Effects of exposure to low level radiofrequency fields on acetylcholine release in hippocampus of freely moving rats. Bioelectromagnetics. May: 23(4):249-55 (2002).

[22] Aalto S, Haarala C, et al. Mobile phone affects cerebral blood flow in humans. Journal of Cerebral Blood Flow Metab. Jul; 26(7):885-90 (2006); Huber R, et al. Exposure to pulse-modulated radio frequency electromagnetic fields affects regional cerebral blood flow. European Journal of Neuroscience, Feb; 21(4):1000-6 (2005).

[23] Lennart Hardell, et al. Pooled analysis of two case–control studies on use of cellular and cordless telephones and the risk for malignant brain tumours diagnosed in 1997–2003. Volume 79, Number 8 / September, 2006; Ken K. Karipidis, et al. Occupational exposure to ionizing and non-ionizing radiation and risk of non-Hodgkin lymphoma. Volume 80, Number 8 / August, 2007. See also Extensive Cell Phone Use Linked To Brain Tumors, Swedish Study, Medical News Today, April 1, 2006 www.medicalnewstoday.com/articles/40764.php.

[24] Frei MR, et al., Chronic exposure of cancer-prone mice to low-level 2450 MHz radiofrequency radiation, Bioelectromagnetics. 1998;19(1):20-31; Frei MR, et al., Chronic, low-level (1.0 W/kg) exposure of mice prone to mammary cancer to 2450 MHz microwaves, Radiat Res. 1998 Nov;150(5):568-76.

[25] Dr. Minoru Inouye, et al., Effect of 2,450 MHz microwave radiation on the development of the rat brain, Teratology, vol. 28, no. 3, pp. 413-419.

The bottom line is that there are conflicting studies out there and the controversies over microwaves will continue.

In my opinion, there are individuals who may be more sensitive to electromagnetic fields and/or radiation than others. There are no tests for this sensitivity that I'm aware of, but if you move out of a highly charged environment, the symptoms do go away quickly and you should notice a difference within a day or so.

In the interest of lowering your toxic burden in this modern world, I would suggest you eliminate your microwave oven, since it's only a convenience (get a Turbo Oven), and minimize your use of a cell phone and any other appliance that may emit radiation. You should also use wired connections for your computer and replace your CRT with a flat-panel monitor.

Reading Labels & Ingredients

The first rule about eating the RAVE Diet is that you should not have to worry about labels because Mother Nature does not have to label her products! And the vast majority of the food you consume should not come with a label. Having said that, it's inevitable you will purchase food that comes in a package, so we need to discuss how to read nutrition labels.

Due to food industry lobbying designed to hide bad ingredients and confuse the customer, you almost have to attend night school to understand food labeling. Let's simplify it.

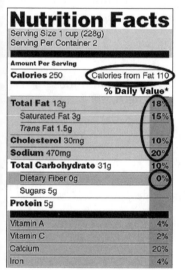

The label to the left is for macaroni and cheese (which you should never eat!). There are three circles you should focus on. The first is "Calories from Fat." Manufacturers rarely do the math for you, but this is 44 percent fat (110 / 250 = .44). Put it back on the shelf. You should ideally find products with less than 10 percent fat.

Next are Total Fat, Saturated Fat and Cholesterol, shown as a percent of daily calories. Look for zeroes. You will find many choices of packaged products with these numbers at health food stores.

After cholesterol is sodium. This is a big item in packaged products because it's used as a preservative and percentages will vary all over the place. The lower, the better.

Look closely at the serving size because the trend is to make serving sizes smaller in order to disguise just how bad a product really is. Many candy bars, for example, are now two servings!

The last circle is Dietary Fiber, which is of great importance. In this case, the larger the number, the better.

A Simple Rule of Thumb About Fat

If you are trying to maintain a diet at 10 percent fat, anything more than one gram of fat per 100 calories is higher than you want. Two grams of fat per 100 calories is 20 percent fat.

Again, due to food industry lobbying, a product can be labeled "fat free" and it can list zero grams of fat, if the fat content is less than 0.5 grams of fat. This is how foods can have oil or high-fat ingredients listed in their Nutrition Facts label, yet contain "zero" fat. Fat free means less than 0.5 grams of fat per serving. Low fat means less than 3 grams of fat per serving.

When food manufacturers moved to fat free packaged goods, what they did in many products was add more sugar and simple (refined) carbohydrates to replace the fat, so instead of *eating* fat, you're quickly *creating* fat inside your body.

Ingredients

On ingredients lists, the top three ingredients to look for are:

Whole, sprouted wheat or organic rolled oats. These should be the first ingredient in any grain product, such as bread or cereal.

Hydrogenated oils – never purchase a product that contains the word "hydrogenated" anywhere in the ingredients.

Sugar, high fructose or fructose, sucrose, glucose, or sorbitol should never be the first, second or third ingredient. In fact, the best products have none of these ingredients.

Also, never purchase anything with the word "instant" on it, such as instant oatmeal.

There will also be a list of ingredients on the package with names most of us could never pronounce. Here is a *short* list of ingredients you should avoid:

all oils, especially hydrogenated oils (partially, fully or whatever)	lactic acid
	lactose
alum (as in aluminum)	lactulose
artificial colorings (any food dye)	lard
BHT	monodiglycerides
calcium propionate	monoglycerides
carrageenan (some are sensitive to this)	monosodium glutamate (MSG)
caseinogen	mycoprotein
casein	palmitate
collagen	polysorbates
diglycerides and monoglycerides	rennet
EDTA	rennin
gelatin	sodium caseinate
glycerin/glycerides	sodium nitrite
hydrolyzed vegetable protein	sugar (any form of sugar)
hydrolyzed oat flour	sulfites
hydrolyzed plant protein	vegetable oils, especially hydrogenated
hydrolysates	oils (partially, fully or whatever)
hydrogenated vegetable oils	whey

A comprehensive list of ingredients would require a book, so in general, if you can't pronounce it, don't put it in your mouth.[1] When in doubt, your best bet is to

---

[1] The latest problem on this front involved "nano food additives," which utilize nanotechnology. Nanotechnology involves the design and manipulation of materials on molecular scales, smaller than the width of a human hair and invisible to the naked eye. These are being introduced into foods without any regulation, at the time of this

166 – Healing Cancer From Inside Out

put the product back on the shelf and go for natural products that come in their natural packages.

Sticky Labels on Fruit

Ever noticed those little "brand" stickers on fruit? They tell you how the product was grown or "created."

There's a number on the label known as the "price look up" or PLU code that speeds up the check out process. But there's more to the PLU than just price.

Conventionally grown produce has a 4-number PLU code.

Genetically engineered produce has a 5-number PLU, beginning with 8.

Organically grown fruit has a 5-number PLU, beginning with 9.

Using this system for an apple, the numbering would look like this:

4011 - conventional grown apple
84011 - genetically engineered apple
94011 - organically grown apple

Organic Labeling

100 Percent Organic: Must contain only organically produced ingredients.
Organic: Defined by the USDA as containing 95 percent of organic ingredients.
Made With Organic: Must contain at least 70 percent organic ingredients. These foods cannot bear the USDA organic seal.
Some Organic Ingredients: Products with less than 70 percent organic ingredients are only allowed to list the organic items in the ingredient panel on the side of the package. These also cannot display the USDA organic seal.

Don't confuse the label "organic" with the label "natural." Natural is a loose term generally meaning that no artificial ingredients were added in processing and has nothing to do with how the product was grown or raised.

What Organic Means

Organic standards require that the land used to grow organic food go through a three year "transition period" to make sure the crops are free of synthetic pesticides and synthetic fertilizers.

All organic agriculture prohibits the use of synthetic pesticides and fertilizers, irradiation and sewage sludge. In addition, no genetically modified organisms can be contained in anything labeled organic.

---

writing, and people are rightly concerned about their safety. Using nanotechnologies in food is estimated to be a $20 billion market by 2010. Again, the best way to avoid such additives is to purchase whole, organic foods.

Organic standards specify that animals may only be fed plant diets, with no animal by-products, which eliminates the risk of certain diseases, such as mad cow disease.

Organic products are also likely to taste better and be free of artificial preservatives and chemicals.

PART 5 – Sample Recipes

The following presents a wide variety of recipes ranging from juicing through breakfast, lunch and dinner – and everything in-between. Some of these recipes were generously supplied by various individuals and organizations and we thank them.[1]

Green Juicing

Green juicing is an excellent way to get concentrated nutrients into your system. The lack of fiber is the trade-off with juicing and because of that, we recommend you juice only once a day. If you do not have a juicer or cannot afford one, you can skip juicing altogether. Or visit your local natural foods store or juice bar and have them make the recipes below.

You can get a basic juicer for $100 to $150. You can also get much more expensive models, such as a Green Star juicer (www.greenstar.com), which actually presses the produce, instead of grinding it. This creates less heat, which increases the juice's quality.

Insofar as directions are concerned, they are the same for all recipes. Cut the ingredients so they will fit into your juicer, juice all ingredients and mix together! If you find the taste too strong, add another carrot or slice of apple.

Green tops, such as the tops of carrots, should always be included in the juicing.

There are an infinite variety of combinations, so please feel free to experiment with different ingredients, depending on what's in the frig!

Cabbage and Celery

3 medium carrots
1 stalk of celery
1/2 green apple
1/4 head of cabbage

Carrot and Cabbage

3-4 Carrots
1-2 Celery stalks
Small wedge cabbage

---

[1] Physicians Committee for Responsible Medicine, Vegetarians in Paradise, Dorit from her book Celebrating Our Raw Nature.

Cabbage, Beet and Kiwis

2 large kiwis
1 beet (with greens)
1/2 head cabbage

Cucumber, Carrot and Beet

3 carrots
1/2 cucumber
1/2 beet with the greens

Garden Variety

6-8 tomatoes
3-4 green onions
2 carrots
2 stalks celery
1/2 green pepper
1/2 bunch spinach
1/2 bunch parsley

Green Soup

1 leaf collard green, chopped
2 stalks celery
1 leaf kale
1 large tomato
2 cloves garlic
2 pieces scallions, chopped
1/4 cup lemon juice, freshly squeezed
1/4 tsp cayenne pepper

Roll garlic in kale and collard leaf and push through juicer hopper with tomato and celery. Pour mixture into a blender. Add lemon juice and mix. Add cayenne pepper. Mix and adjust to taste. Serve with chopped scallion sprinkled on top of soup.

Renewal

8 large carrots
5 celery stalks
5 radishes
1 large green apple
1 cup cranberries
1/2 large beet
1/2 turnip
1/2 parsnip
1/4 rutabaga
1/8 head red cabbage

Spinach and Celery Delight

4 large spinach leaves
3 stalks celery
2 large carrots
1/2 cup parsley
1/2 beet root
1/2 cup alfalfa sprouts

Spinach, Celery and Asparagus

3 celery stalks
2 asparagus stalks
1 large tomato
Handful of spinach

Sky High Veggies

6 Brussels sprouts
4 medium sweet potatoes (without skin)
4 medium carrots
1 broccoli stalk
1 garlic clove pressed
1 cucumber

The Ultimate

3 carrots
3 collard leaves
2 celery stalks
2 beets
2 garlic cloves
1 turnip
1/2 bunch spinach
1/2 head cabbage
1/2 onion
1/4 bunch parsley

Tomato Juice #1
  (can also be blended)

6 tomatoes
1 cup beet leaves, chopped
1 slice lemon

Tomato Juice #2
  (can also be blended)

4 ripe tomatoes
1 cup green lettuce, packed

V-11 Juice

3 stalks of celery
2 kale leaves
1 head of romaine lettuce
1 cucumber
1 green apple
1 handful cilantro or parsley
1 handful of fennel (use stalk as well)
1 clove garlic
1-2 carrots
1/4 papaya
Handful of spinach leaves

Green Blending (smoothies)

Green blending (smoothies) is an excellent and easy ways to get more green vegetables into your diet. The basic difference between blending and juicing is that you keep everything in foods when you blend them, particularly the fiber, which is extremely important when fighting cancer.

The recipes below are simply suggestions. Feel free to substitute or add ingredients, depending on what you have handy. You can easily adjust smoothies to suit your taste as well. After they are blended, taste a little and if it isn't right, add more ingredients. Smoothies are an excellent way to start the day.

Most ordinary blenders should do the job, but if they don't you can get a very good high-speed blender for less than $100. Vita-Mix is the top of the line and if you get into smoothies, you may want to invest in one of these, or a comparable blender, such as Blendtec.

The directions are the same for all smoothies: simply throw everything into the blender (some ingredients will have to be peeled, of course) and blend until smooth.

Smoothie #1

10 mint leaves
2 cups spinach
3 bananas
2 tbsp carob powder (optional)
1 tsp ground flaxseed
1 cup water

Smoothie #2

2 stalks of celery
2 bananas
2 pears
1 green apple
1 handful spinach
1 tsp ground flaxseed
1 cup water

Smoothie #3

1 handful collard green leaves
1 kale leaf
1 handful mint

4 bananas
1 tsp ground flaxseed
1/2 cup water

Smoothie #4

5 kale leaves
4 apples
1 tsp ground flaxseed
1/2 lemon juiced
1/2 cup water (or to taste)

Smoothie #5

2 cups arugula
2 mangoes
1 handful of spinach
1 tsp ground flaxseed
1 cup water

Smoothie #6

6 kale leaves
3 large bananas
1 handful chard leaves
1 tsp ground flaxseed
1 cup water

Smoothie #7

1 pink grapefruit
1 cucumber
1 lime
1 slice pineapple
1 tsp ground flaxseed
1/2 bunch cilantro
Pinch of cinnamon

Smoothie #8

5 mustard green leaves
2 celery sticks
1 tsp ground flaxseed
1/2 lime juiced
1/2 red onion
1/4 bunch of fresh basil
2 cups of water

Smoothie #9

5 kale leaves
3 cloves garlic
1 cup tomatoes
1 tsp ground flaxseed
1/2 bunch dill
1/2 lime juice
2 cups of water

Smoothie #10

5 kale leaves
3 apples
1 tsp ground flaxseed
1/2 lemon juiced

2 cups of water

Smoothie #11

3 cups red grapes
2 handfuls baby Spinach
1 handful parsley
1 tsp ground flaxseed
2 cups of water

Smoothie #12

3 large handfuls baby spinach
3 bananas
1 tsp ground flaxseed
2 cups of water

Smoothie #13

4 large bananas
2 large handfuls of kale
1 small handful of parsley
1 handful of baby spinach
1 tsp ground flaxseed
2 cups of water

Smoothie #14

2 handfuls baby spinach
1 celery stalk
1 handful parsley
1 Granny Smith apple
1/4 tsp ginger powder (or better 1/2 inch ginger)
1 tsp ground flaxseed
2 cups water

Smoothie #15

4 large ripe bananas
2 large handfuls of kale
1 small handful of parsley
1 handful of baby spinach
1 tsp ground flaxseed
2 cups of water

Smoothie #16

2 pears
2 celery stalks
1 cucumber
1 lemon
1 cup spinach
1 tsp ground flaxseed
1/2 inch ginger
1 cup water

Smoothie #17

1 bunch bok choy

1 banana
1 pear
2 celery stalks
1 tsp ground flaxseed
1 1/2 cup water

Smoothie #18

2 stalks collard greens
1 piece ginger
1 stalk celery
1/2 pineapple (or 1 pear or 1 apple)
1/2 bunch cilantro

Smoothie #19

2 leaves collard greens
2 stalks celery
1 tomato
2 cloves garlic
1 green apple

Fast Food: Meals in Minutes

Most of us come home from work and the last thing we want to do is cook a meal. For myself, I usually open the refrigerator or pantry door and see what I have on-hand, then prepare a quick meal.

If this is you, one of the best ways to eat is to open your freezer door and "pour" out a meal using frozen vegetables. Frozen vegetables are almost as good as fresh and sometimes better (in terms of nutrients) because they're often picked and processed at their peak of ripeness, using techniques that lock in a slew of nutrients. They're also better than canned because most don't have added sodium. Any grocery store will have bags of frozen vegetables you can use. Make sure they are organic.

Just pour them into a bowl, stir-fry them together. Add spices or stir in some tomato sauce with spices and Voila! You have a meal in minutes.

What about work? Again, think frozen. Just pour some vegetables into a container and take it to work. By lunchtime, the vegetables are pretty much thawed. Heat it up at work and you have lunch.

I usually cut up a head of romaine lettuce, for example, put it in a bag and keep it in the frig. This way, I can create a salad in minutes. And, don't forget, you can always visit your local salad bar on the way home from work.

I sometimes make a big pot of brown rice every week. Use it as the base and pour frozen vegetables into it. Add tomato or another sauce, stir it up and you have your lunch in minutes.

If you're on the go and like fast meals, you should set aside some time on the weekend to cook large amounts and then refrigerate or freeze it in serving sizes appropriate for your appetite. The idea is not that you eat the same meal seven days in a row, but that you build a supply of various meals. This will work like magic and you'll spend far less time preparing large meals to re-heat and last through the week than you would preparing separate, individual meals.

Here are a few samples. It's not the foods used below, as much as the technique because you can substitute any foods for a quick meal, depending on what you have in the refrigerator or pantry.

3-Step Quickie

1) Cut up assorted vegetables and sauté or stir-fry them in water or a vegetable broth. Cook over medium heat.

2) Stir in your favorite seasonings and sauce (e.g., tomato sauce, black bean sauce, curry, Thai sauce, etc. See *Seasonings* and *Sauces*).

3) Serve on a bed of your favorite food, like brown rice or sweet potatoes.

Rice, Beans & Vegetables

Brown rice in the bottom of the bowl (rice usually prepared beforehand in large quantities).

When finished, add raw or steamed vegetables and beans.

Mix-in any tomato or other sauce for flavoring, along with herbs and spices and heat it in a pan.

Any and All Vegetable Soup

Cut up your favorite vegetables in large quantities. Put them all in a pot full of water (large enough to handle your vegetables).

Add your favorite herbs, spices and sauces.

Cook until done. (Note that crock-pots or pressure cookers are ideal for this.)

This will last for days or longer and can stored in the refrigerator or freezer.

When ready to eat, just heat it up and serve.

Keeping Brown Rice

I usually prepare a large quantity of brown rice using a rice cooker. This is a great investment because it takes me literally two minutes to prepare the rice and when it's done, the cooker goes into automatic warmer mode so I don't have to watch over it.

Just add the brown rice and twice the amount of water, e.g., 1 cup rice = 2 cups water.

Add seasonings to taste.

Press the appropriate buttons and you're done.

Rice can be stored in the refrigerator. It will cake and stick together, but will be fine once you heat it up again in a small amount of water.

Breakfast Guidelines

When preparing breakfast, be your own chef. If you don't particularly like the texture of rolled oats, for example, mix-in Grape-Nuts with them and have your very own designer-breakfast the way you like it. Instead of using jellies and jams, try spreading whole fruits on toast, such as a banana.

Anything "instant," such as instant oatmeal, should be put back on the shelf.

Here are some general suggestions:

Oatmeal with fruit and whole wheat bread
Whole grain cereal with raisins, bananas, ground flaxseed
Green smoothie (see *Green Blending*)
Buckwheat, oat flour and flaxseed pancakes

Cereals

Below are some of the more popular cereal brands, which contain whole grains. Be sure to inspect the ingredients list as food manufacturers change ingredients over time. (See *Reading Labels & Ingredients*.) Use water only to moisten these cereals to taste.

Whole grains - Cold
Arrowhead Mills Organic Amaranth Flakes
Erewhon Crispy Brown Rice (like Rice Krispies)
Grape-Nuts (not flakes)
Health Valley Organic Fiber 7 Multigrain flakes
Heart-To-Heart (Kashi)
Nature's Path Organic Cereals
Puffed Wheat
Quaker Old-Fashioned (rolled) Oats (not instant)
Shredded wheat

Whole grains - Hot

Bulgar cereal mix
Oat bran
Oatmeal (never buy instant oatmeal)
Quaker Multigrain
Quaker Old-Fashioned (rolled) Oats (not instant)
Ralston High Fiber
Roman Meal
Steel-cut Oats (the best oatmeal)
Wheatena

Breakfast Recipes

Black Beans with Salsa on Toast
Serves 2

1 cup dry black beans
1/4 cup diced onions
1 tsp thinly sliced jalapenos
1 large tomato, diced
1 garlic clove pressed
4 slices of your favorite toast or tortillas

Heat and mash beans (*See Rules for Meal Preparation, Bean Preparation*). For the salsa, mix the jalapenos, tomatoes, and onions, adjusting amounts to taste. Serve the beans and salsa on toast or with tortillas.

Bulgar Breakfast Cereal

2/3 cups bulgur
1 1/3 cups cold water
dried fruit of choice (raisins, apricots, papaya)
favorite spices (e.g., cinnamon, nutmeg)
brown rice or maple syrup

Add bulgur to cold water, bring to a boil, and then down to a simmer. Simmer in a covered pan for 12-15 minutes. Should be moist like oatmeal. Add dried fruit, spices and syrup to taste.

French Toast
Serves 2 to 3

2 medium bananas
2/3 cup water
2 tbsp maple syrup
1/8 tsp ground cinnamon
4 slices bread

Blend bananas, water, maple syrup, and cinnamon until smooth. Pour into a flat, shallow dish and soak bread slices 1 minute on each side. Transfer carefully to a skillet. Cook first side until lightly browned, about 3 minutes, then turn and cook second side until browned. Serve with fresh fruit.

Granola – Maple Walnut
Makes about 6 cups

3 cups rolled oats
1 cup wheat germ
1/2 cup chopped walnuts
1/2 cup raisins
1/4 cup sesame seeds
1/4 cup maple syrup
2 tbsp molasses
1 tsp cinnamon

Preheat oven to 300. Combine all ingredients in a large bowl and mix thoroughly. Transfer to a 9 × 13-inch baking dish. Bake, turning often with a spatula, until mixture is golden brown, about 25 minutes.

Muesli
Makes 3 cups

2 cups rolled oats
1/2 cup chopped dried fruit (apples, figs, apricots, etc.)
1/2 cup raisins

Combine all ingredients. They may be left whole or ground in a food processor until they are of a fairly fine, uniform texture. Store in an airtight container in the refrigerator. Serve with water to moisten and fresh cut fruit toppings.

Pancakes – Cornmeal
Makes 16 3-inch pancakes

1 cup water
1/2 cup cornmeal
1/2 cup whole wheat pastry flour
2 tbsp maple syrup
1 tbsp cider vinegar
1/2 tsp sodium-free baking powder
1/4 tsp baking soda

In a large bowl mix water, maple syrup, and vinegar. Set aside. In separate bowl stir together cornmeal, flour, baking powder, baking soda. Add to water mixture, stirring to remove any lumps and make a batter. Add more water if batter seems too thick. On skillet or griddle, pour small amounts of batter onto the heated surface and cook until tops bubble. Turn carefully with a spatula and cook the second sides until browned. Use fresh fruit, or maple syrup for serving

Pancakes – Old-Fashioned
Makes 16 3-inch pancakes

1 ripe banana, mashed
1 cup water
1/2 cup buckwheat flour
1/2 cup cornmeal
2 tbsp maple syrup
1 tbsp vinegar
1/2 tsp sodium-free baking powder
1/4 tsp baking soda

Mix buckwheat flour, cornmeal, baking powder, baking soda. In a large bowl, combine mashed banana, maple syrup, vinegar, and water. Add flour mixture, stirring just enough to remove any lumps and make a batter. Add more water if batter seems too thick. On skillet or griddle, pour small amounts of batter onto the heated surface and cook until tops bubble. Turn carefully with a spatula and cook the second sides until browned. Use fresh fruit, or maple syrup for serving

Quinoa Cereal
Makes one large serving

1/2 cup water
1/4 cup quinoa
1/4 cup steel cut oats
1/4 cup crushed pinapple or pineapple juice
1 tsp blackstrap mollasses
        currants or raisins to taste

Boil then simmer the quinoa in water and molasses for ten minutes. Add the oats and fruit and simmer for another 15 minutes.

Rolled Oats Cold

Rolled oats (not cooked)
Banana (or peach, mango, kiwis, melons, apricots, etc.)
Mixed berries
Pineapple slices
Raisins
1 tbsp ground flaxseed
Moisten with water (to taste)

Pour rolled oats into bowl. Add flaxseed and water.

Sweet Potato Breakfast
Makes four servings

2 baked sweet potatoes
2 bananas, sliced
1 apple, peeled, cored, and diced
1/2 tsp cinnamon
1/4 blackstrap molasses

Mash the sweet potatoes. Mix in bananas. Sprinkle with cinnamon and molasses.

Waffles – Oatmeal
Makes 6 waffles

1 banana
2 cups rolled oats
2 cups water
1 tbsp maple syrup
1 tsp vanilla

Preheat waffle iron to medium-high. Combine oats, water, banana, maple syrup and vanilla in a blender. Blend on high speed until completely smooth. Pour in batter and cook until golden brown (5-10 minutes without lifting lid.) Serve with fresh fruit.

Whole Wheat Pancakes
Makes 24 2-inch pancakes

1 banana
1 1/4 cups water
1 cup whole wheat pastry flour or whole wheat flour
1 tbsp maple syrup
2 tsp sodium-free baking powder

In a large bowl, mash banana, then stir in water and maple syrup. In a separate bowl mix flour and baking powder. Add to banana mixture and stir until smooth. Pour small amounts of batter onto a preheated griddle or skillet with a small amount of oil substitute and cook until tops bubble. Flip with a spatula and cook second side until golden brown, about 1 minute. Use fresh fruit, or maple syrup for serving

Lunch or Dinner Recipes

Suggestions for Lunch/Dinner

The following are simply suggestions that you can whip up on your own without following any recipe.

Acorn squash with rice
Angel hair zucchini with tomato sauce and sweet potato or squash
Bean soup and stir-fried vegetables
Bean, vegetable and barley soup
Beets, raisins and carrots
Brown rice and vegetables
Carrot soup
Corn chowder
Corn stew
Garden salad
Garden salad wrap
Green beans and garlic mashed sweet potatoes
Lentil, tomato, etc. soup with whole wheat bread
Pasta, tomato sauce and vegetables
Pasta and vegetables
Pasta, tomato sauce and vegetables
Portobello mushroom burgers and beans
Raw vegetables
Rice and vegetables
Roasted eggplant, corn & zucchini wrap
Roasted peppers stuffed with rice and vegetables
Salad stuffed whole wheat pita
Salad and raw vegetables
Stir-fry vegetables
Vegetable soup
Vegetable pate sandwich

Salads – The Main Meal

For dressings, see *Rules for Meal Preparation – Salad Dressings Without Oil*

Salad - Antipasto
Makes about 6 cups

1 large red potato, scrubbed
1 carrot, sliced
1 cup Italian green beans, fresh or frozen
1 cup cauliflower florets
1 small red bell pepper, sliced or diced
2 garlic cloves, pressed
2 tbsp finely chopped parsley
2 tbsp balsamic vinegar
1 tbsp seasoned rice vinegar
1 tbsp vegetable broth
1 tbsp lemon juice
2 tsp apple juice concentrate
1 tsp stone ground or Dijon-style mustard
1/4 tsp black pepper

Dice potatoes and steam with carrots over boiling water until just tender, about 10 minutes. Place in a salad bowl. Steam green beans and cauliflower until just tender. Add to salad. Add bell pepper and parsley. Mix vinegars, vegetable broth, lemon juice, apple juice concentrate, garlic, mustard and pepper in a small bowl. Pour over vegetables, and toss to mix.

Salad – Aztec
Makes about 8 cups

3 cups dry black beans (*See Rules for Meal Preparation, Bean Preparation*)
2 tomatoes, diced
2 garlic cloves, pressed or finely minced
1 lemon or lime, juiced
1 10-ounce bag frozen corn, thawed, or 2 cups fresh corn
3/4 cup chopped fresh cilantro (optional)
1/2 cup finely chopped red onion
1 green bell pepper, seeded and diced
1 red or yellow bell pepper, seeded and diced
2 tbsp rice vinegar
2 tbsp apple cider or distilled vinegar
2 tsp ground cumin
1 tsp coriander
1/2 tsp red pepper flakes or a pinch of cayenne

In a large bowl, combine beans, onion, bell peppers, corn, tomatoes, and cilantro. In a small bowl, whisk together vinegars, lemon juice, garlic, cumin, coriander, and red pepper flakes. Pour over salad and toss gently to mix.

Salad – Bean Salad
Serves 10

(*See Rules for Meal Preparation, Bean Preparation*)
2 cups dry kidney beans
2 cups pinto beans
2 cups black-eyed peas
2 cups frozen baby lima beans, thawed
1 cup frozen corn, thawed
1 large red bell pepper, diced
1/2 medium red onion, finely diced

Toss all ingredients together. Serve cold or at room temperature.

Salad – Black Bean & Corn

3 cups dry black beans (*See Rules for Meal Preparation, Bean Preparation*)
2 cups frozen corn kernels, thawed
2 tomatoes, chopped
1 red pepper, chopped
1 jalapeno pepper, minced
1 cup chopped green onions
1/2 cup chopped red onion
1/2 cup chopped cilantro
1-2 tbsp juice from 1 lime
1 tbsp vegetable broth
1 tsp minced garlic

Combine first seven ingredients in a large bowl. Make dressing with lime juice, cilantro, garlic, pepper and vegetable broth. Combine well. Pour over salad ingredients and toss lightly to combine. Chill several hours before serving.

Salad – Black-eyed Peas Salad
Makes about 5 cups

2 cups cooked black-eyed peas
1-1/2 cups cooked brown rice
1 celery stalk, thinly sliced (about 1/2 cup)
1 tomato, diced
1/2 cup finely sliced green onions
2 tbsp finely chopped parsley

Combine the above ingredients in a mixing bowl. Add no-oil salad dressing.

Salad – Broccoli
Makes about 4 cups

1 bunch broccoli
1–2 garlic cloves, minced
1/2 cup finely sliced red onion
1/2 cup seasoned rice vinegar
1 tbsp vegetable broth
1 tsp teriyaki sauce
1/2 tsp dried red pepper flakes

Cut or break broccoli into small florets. Transfer to a salad bowl. Add remaining ingredients and toss to mix. Chill, tossing once or twice, for 20 minutes or longer before serving.

Salad – Brussels Sprout-White Bean

1/2 pound Brussels sprouts, ends removed and halved
4 cups dry Great Northern white beans (*See Rules for Meal Preparation, Bean Preparation*)
2/3 cup Italian olives, depitted and halved
1 cup red onions, sliced into thin strips
1 clove garlic, minced
2 tbsp water
1 tbsp apple cider vinegar
4 tsp celery juice
2 tsp sage, chopped
1 1/2 tbsp lemon zest
1 tsp maple syrup
Pinch cayenne pepper

Steam Brussels sprouts for a short time so they are still crispy. Add all ingredients to a large salad bowl. Toss and serve or allow to marinate for 1-3 hours before serving.

Salad – Chinese Cabbage & Walnut
Serves 4

1 head Chinese cabbage
1 cup carrots, grated
1/2 cup walnuts, chopped
1 yellow bell pepper
1 tbsp apple cider vinegar
Herb seasonings of choice (to taste)

Salad – Colorful
Serves 4

1 sweet red pepper, cut into chunks
1 orange
1 cup of snap peas, cut in half
1 cucumber, peeled and cut into chunks
8 fresh basil leaves, sliced
1 tbsp seasoned rice vinegar
cracked black pepper, to taste

Remove the peel off the orange and cut the peeled fruit into bite size chunks. In medium bowl, mix together the orange, red pepper, cucumber, and basil. Sprinkle with rice vinegar and season with pepper. Toss and serve.

Salad – Crunchy
Serves 6

1 15-ounce can diced beets, drained
2 medium-size carrots, peeled and cut into thin strips or diced
1 small jicama, peeled and cut into thin strips or diced
3 tbsp of lemon juice
2 tbsp seasoned rice vinegar
2 tsp stone ground mustard
1/2 tsp dried dill weed

Place beet cubes into a large salad bowl, along with jicama and carrot pieces. In a small bowl, mix lemon juice, vinegar, mustard, and dill; pour over the salad. Toss to mix. Serve warm or chilled.

Salad – Cucumber Arame
Serves 4 to 6

1 cucumber
1 cup arame
1 cup water
2 tbsp lemon juice
2 tbsp water
1 tbsp brown rice vinegar
1 tsp low-sodium Tamari (soy sauce)

Peel and halve the cucumber lengthwise. Transfer to a bowl and let stand 15 minutes. Drain thoroughly. Meanwhile, soak the arame in one cup of water until soft, 10 to 15 minutes. Mix together lemon juice, Tamari, vinegar and 2 tablespoons of water to make dressing. Drain any excess water from arame, then combine with cucumber and dressing.

Salad – Cucumber, Mango & Spinach
Serves 10-12

1 bag or bunch of spinach
1 mango, peeled and cut into bite size pieces
1 large English cucumber, peeled and sliced
6 scallions, thinly sliced
1/2 cup fresh, chopped basil leaves
Juice of 1 lime
1/2 cup seasoned rice vinegar
Fresh cracked black pepper to taste

Wash and drain spinach, tear into bite-sized pieces if necessary, and put into a large serving bowl. Toss mango, cucumber, scallions, and basil in a medium bowl. Dress with lime juice and vinegar. Arrange mango mixture on spinach and sprinkle with fresh cracked black pepper.

Salad – Fiesta
Serves 10

4 cups dry black beans (*See Rules for Meal Preparation, Bean Preparation*)
2 cups frozen corn, thawed
2 large tomatoes, diced
1 large green bell pepper, diced
1 large red or yellow bell pepper, diced
3/4 cups chopped cilantro
1/2 cup chopped red onion

Combine beans with the corn, tomatoes, bell peppers, red onion, and cilantro. Toss with no-oil dressing.

Salad – Mediterranean Rice Salad
Serves 6 to 8

3 Roma tomatoes, cut into chunks
3 cups cooked brown rice
1 green pepper, chopped
1 cucumber, peeled and cut into chunks
1 cup green beans, broken into small pieces, blanched or raw
1/2 cup fresh basil leaves, sliced
1/2 cup seasoned rice vinegar
1 tbsp mustard
1 tbsp vegetable broth
1/2 tsp dried parsley flakes
juice of 1 lemon

In medium bowl, mix together rice, pepper, green beans, cucumber, tomato, and basil. Stir together mustard, rice vinegar, lemon juice, vegetable broth, and parsley. Pour over salad and toss to mix. Season with pepper. Toss and serve.

Salad – Minty Purslane Salad
Serves 2 to 4

1 head romaine, washed, dried and torn into small pieces
1 med cucumber, diced
2 large firm tomatoes, diced
4 green onions, chopped
1 green bell pepper, seeded and chopped
1 cup purslane, chopped
1/2 cup arugula or watercress leaves, chopped
1/4 cup fresh flat-leaf parsley, chopped
1/4 cup fresh mint, chopped

Mix together with dressing and serve.

Salad – Mixed Greens with Apples & Walnuts
Makes about 4 cups

6 cups salad mix or washed and torn butter lettuce
1 tart green apple (Granny Smith, pippin, or similar)
1/4 cup chopped walnuts
3-4 tbsp seasoned rice vinegar

Place salad mix or torn leaf lettuce into a bowl. Core and dice apple and add to salad along with walnuts. Sprinkle with seasoned rice vinegar and toss to mix.

Salad – Pasta Salad
Serves 8-10

12 ounces pasta shells (about 2 cups)
1 jar water-packed artichoke hearts, drained and quartered
2-3 cups button mushrooms (about 1/2 pound)
1 garlic clove
1 small red bell pepper, diced
1/2 cup chopped green onions
1/3 cup seasoned rice vinegar
1/4 cup cider vinegar
3 tbsp water
3 tbsp chopped fresh parsley
2 tbsp fresh lemon juice (optional)
2 tsp stone-ground or Dijon-style mustard
1/2 tsp each dried basil and oregano
1/4 tsp black pepper

Cook until pasta is tender. Rinse, drain, place in a large bowl. Add artichoke hearts and mushrooms. In a blender, combine the vinegars, lemon juice, mustard, 1/4 cup green onions, garlic, seasonings, and water. Process until smooth. Pour over pasta, and allow to marinate until pasta is cool. Add the remaining green onions, parsley, and red bell pepper and gently toss to mix.

Salad – Rice Salad

3 cups cooked brown rice
3 Roma tomatoes, cut into chunks
1 green, yellow or red pepper, chopped
1 cucumber, peeled and cut into chunks
1 cup raw green beans, cut into small pieces
1/2 cup basil leaves, sliced
1/2 cup seasoned rice vinegar
1 tbsp mustard
1/2 tsp dried parsley flakes
1/2 tsp Italian seasoning
juice of 1 lemon

In bowl, mix together rice, pepper, green beans, cucumber, tomato, and basil. Stir together mustard, rice vinegar, lemon juice and parsley. Pour over salad and toss to mix. Season with pepper and Tabasco (optional) to taste. Toss and serve.

Salad – Spanish Wild Rice

2 cups wild rice
Dried apricots, diced
Walnuts, chopped
Juice from one orange, freshly squeezed
Spring onions, chopped
Balsamic vinegar

Cook rice until done, but still a little firm. Toss in some dried apricots, walnuts and spring onions. Pour Balsamic vinegar to taste over the rice and chill.

Salad – Spinach
Serves 2

2 cups spinach
1/2 cup sliced mushrooms
1/4 cup chopped green onions
Tamari (optional)
Sesame seeds, for garnish

Thoroughly wash the spinach, tearing the larger leaves. Drain well. Add the mushrooms and green onions, and toss well. Sprinkle with Tamari, if desired, and then sprinkle each serving with sesame seeds.

Salad – Spinach with Fruit
Serves 4

4 cups cleaned spinach leaves
2 oranges, peeled, sliced, and quartered
1 cucumber, peeled, sliced and quartered
1 sweet red pepper, seeded and chopped
2 tbsp raw or roasted sunflower seeds

Toss spinach with cucumber, orange, and red pepper chunks in medium sized bowl. Sprinkle with sunflower seeds. Serve with no-oil dressing on the side.

Salad – Squash, Corn & Bean Salad
Makes about 8 cups

15-ounces fresh or frozen corn
2 cups black beans (*See Rules for Meal Preparation, Bean Preparation*)
1 red bell pepper, diced
2 cups butternut or kabocha squash, julienne or cut into 1/4-inch cubes (available frozen in health food stores)
1 cup jicama, julienne or cut into 1/4-inch cubes
1/2 cup red onion
1/2 cup chopped cilantro
1/4 cup pumpkin seeds
1/4 cup seasoned rice vinegar
2 tbsp lemon or lime juice
1 tsp each: cumin, coriander, chili powder
1 garlic clove, pressed or minced

Combine squash, jicama, bell pepper, corn, beans, onion, cilantro and pumpkin seeds in a large bowl. Mix vinegar, lemon juice, cumin, coriander, chili powder and garlic. Pour over salad and toss to mix.

Salad – String Bean
Serves 3

1 pound string beans
2 cloves garlic, minced
1 onion, diced
1 tbsp water
1 cup water
1 tsp her seasoning of choice
1tsp tamari

Steam beans until soft. Sauté garlic and onion in small frying pan using water and tamari. In a bowl, mix water and remaining ingredients. Put beans in bowl and add all ingredients and mix. Serve chilled.

Salad – Stuffed Tomato
Serves 5

5 large ripe tomatoes
2 cups dry garbanzo beans (*See Rules for Meal Preparation, Bean Preparation*)
1 stalk celery, chopped (optional)

Scoop out tomatoes, saving pulp for a sauce. Fill tomatoes with beans and celery. Season with pepper. Garnish with sauce and lettuce or sprouts.

Salad – Three Bean
Serves 4

(*See Rules for Meal Preparation, Bean Preparation*)
2 cups dry kidney beans
2 cups dry garbanzo beans
2 cups dry lima beans
1 cup onion, chopped
1/2 cup green pepper, chopped
4 tsp vegetable broth

Toss ingredients together. Serve hot or cold with a grain or bread. To serve cold for a salad, add a few drops of lemon juice or vinegar.

Salad – Tomato, Cucumber & Basil
Serves 6

4 fresh tomatoes, quartered and sliced
1/2 large English cucumber, peeled, quartered and sliced
1/2 cup fresh basil leaves,
3-4 tbsp balsamic vinegar

Arrange cucumber and tomato in a flat bowl. Add basil leaves, dress with balsamic vinegar, and sprinkle with fresh cracked black pepper.

Salad – White Bean
Makes about 2 1/2 cups

2 cups dry white beans (*See Rules for Meal Preparation, Bean Preparation*)
1 small red bell pepper, diced
1/2 cup finely chopped fresh parsley
1 lemon, juiced
2 tsp balsamic vinegar
1/4 tsp garlic granules or powder
1/4 tsp black pepper

Combine all ingredients in a large bowl and toss to mix. Let stand 10 to 15 minutes before serving.

Soups & Stews

Chowder – Kale and Rice
Serves 6

2 cups, diced stewed tomatoes
2 cups vegetable broth
2 cups chopped kale
2 cups dry garbanzo beans (*See Rules for Meal Preparation, Bean Preparation*)
1 cup cooked brown rice
1 cup chopped onion
1 cup chopped red bell pepper
1 1/2 cups water
1/2 cup chopped leeks
1/3 cup sliced almonds
1 tbsp paprika
2 tsp vegetable broth for sautéing
2 bay leaves

Heat the broth over medium-high heat. Add the onion, pepper, leeks, and almonds. Sauté for 2 minutes. Add the almonds, paprika, bay leaves, water, tomatoes, and broth. Bring to boil. Add the kale, rice, and garbanzo beans. Reduce heat and simmer 10 minutes, or until thoroughly heated.

Soup – Black Bean Creamy
Serves 4 to 6

3 cloves garlic, crushed
6-7 cups water
2-1/2 cups dry black beans
1 cup water
1 tbsp vegetable broth
tortillas for garnish (whole wheat)
lettuce for garnish

Soak beans overnight. Drain and cover with water. Add the garlic and cook until soft, about 2 hours, or five minutes in a pressure cooker. Blend beans with the cooking water and return to pot. Reheat with vegetable broth and water. Garnish with thinly sliced fried tortillas and strips of lettuce.

Soup – Carrot and Red Pepper
Serves 4

6 carrots, thinly sliced
2 red bell peppers, roasted
1 onion, chopped
2 cups water
2 cups water or vegetable stock
2 tsp lemon juice
2 tsp balsamic vinegar
1/4 tsp freshly ground black pepper

Place the chopped onion and carrots into a pot with the water and simmer, covered, over medium heat until the carrots can be easily pierced with a fork, about 20 minutes. Roast the peppers by placing them over an open gas flame or directly under the broiler. Place in a bowl, cover, and let stand about 15 minutes. Cut the peppers in half and remove the seeds. Blend the carrot mixture along with the peppers in several small batches. Add some of the water to each batch to facilitate blending. Return to the pot and add the lemon juice, vinegar and pepper. Heat until steamy.

Soup - Cauliflower

2 med. heads of cauliflower
2 stalks of celery
1 leak
1 onion
1 cup brown rice
4 cups vegetable broth
4 water

Separate flowers from cauliflower head. Chop the other vegetables, including the remainder of the cauliflower, into bite sized chunks. Put vegetables, rice and broth in a large soup pot and simmer for 45 minutes (rice and vegetables should be tender). Puree everything in a blender or food processor and serve.

Soup – Chilled Cucumber-Dill
Makes 1 serving

1-1/2 cups water
1/2 cucumber
1 tbsp fresh dill weed or 1 tsp dried dill weed

Chill the water in the freezer for 15 minutes. Put the cucumber through a juicer. Combine the cucumber juice and water in a blender. Pour into a bowl and top with the dill weed.

Soup – Cream of Asparagus
Makes about 7 cups

2 medium-size white potatoes, diced
1 medium-size bunch asparagus (about 4 cups chopped)
2 cups water
2 cups shredded cabbage
1-2 cups water
1 cup (loosely packed) chopped fresh parsley
1/4 cup chopped fresh basil

Dice potatoes (do not peel them). Place them into a large pot with the water. Bring to a simmer, cover and cook until tender. Remove the tough ends from the asparagus, then break stalks into 1- to 2-inch lengths. When potatoes are tender, add asparagus along with cabbage, parsley, and basil. Cover and simmer for about 5 minutes, or until asparagus is just tender when pierced with a fork. In a blender purée the vegetables with cooking liquid, in 2 or 3 batches. Add enough of the water to each batch to facilitate blending. After puréeing all vegetables, pour soup into the pan, then heat gently until steamy.

Soup – Creamy Beet
Makes about 3 cups

1 15-ounce can diced beets
1 cup water
2 tbsp apple juice concentrate
1 tsp balsamic vinegar
1/2 tsp dried dill weed

Place diced beets, water, apple juice concentrate, vinegar, and dill weed into blender. Blend on high speed until completely smooth. Transfer to a medium saucepan and heat gently until steamy. Serve hot or cold.

Soup – Curried Potato and Onion
Serves 6

2 medium onions, chopped
2 large garlic cloves, pressed or minced
4-1/2 cups vegetable broth or bouillon
2 to 3 cups peeled and diced potatoes
3/4 cup water
2 tsp vegetable broth
1-1/2 tsp ground cumin
1-1/2 tsp curry powder, or to taste
1 tsp ground tumeric
chopped fresh chives or cilantro for garnish

In a large soup pot, sauté the garlic and onion in the broth until transparent. Add spices and 1/4 cup broth; stir well and cook for 5 minutes. Add the potatoes and remaining broth. Simmer gently for 20 minutes, or until potatoes are soft. Purée in batches in a food processor or use a hand held blender and blend until smooth. If serving cold, refrigerate for at least 6 hours.

Soup – Curried Sweet Potato
Serves 6

5 cups cubed, peeled sweet potato
4 cups vegetable broth
1 cup chopped onion
1 cup water
1/8 cup vegetable broth
2 tsp curry powder
minced cilantro (optional)

Heat broth in a large saucepan over medium heat. Add the onion and curry powder and sauté for 2 minutes. Add the water, broth, and sweet potatoes. Cook for 30 minutes, or until the sweet potatoes are tender. Place one-third of the sweet potato mixture in a blender and process until smooth. Repeat the procedure with the remaining sweet potato mixture in batches. Return the puréed mixture to the saucepan. Bring the soup to a boil and remove from heat. Garnish with cilantro, if desired.

Soup – Gazpacho
Serves 4

1 plum tomato, seeded and finely diced
2 garlic cloves, chopped
2 cups tomato juice
1/4 cup seeded and diced cucumber
1/4 cup finely diced green bell pepper
1/4 cup red onion, finely diced
1/4 cup zucchini, finely diced (optional)
4 tbs. vegetable broth
2 tbs. bread crumbs
1 tbs. white wine vinegar

Place the tomato juice, garlic and broth in a blender and process until the garlic is puréed. Add the bread crumbs and vinegar, and blend to combine. Add favorite seasonings. Pour into a covered container and chill well, from 2 hours to overnight. When ready to serve, check the seasoning and adjust if necessary. Divide the soup among 4 serving bowls. Add 1 Tbs. each of the diced cucumber, pepper, tomato and onion, plus the zucchini if desired.

Soup – Lentil
Serves 8

2 onions, halved and sliced
4 cloves garlic, minced
3 parsnips, peeled and sliced
10 cups water
5 cups packed chopped dandelion greens or kale
2 cups red lentils, rinsed and drained
1/8 cup vegetable broth
1 5 ounce can tomato paste
3 tbsp chopped parsley, divided
1 tsp dried oregano
1 tsp dried basil
1 tsp black pepper

In a large pot, heat vegetable broth over medium-high heat. Add onions and sauté for 3 minutes. Add garlic and sauté 1 minute more. Add water, lentils, tomato paste, parsnips, 1 tablespoon parsley, oregano, basil, and pepper. Bring to a boil. Reduce heat to low, cover and simmer for 30 minutes. Add dandelion greens and simmer an additional 15 minutes or until greens are soft. Garnish with remaining parsley.

Soup – Lentils with Cabbage
Serves 4 to 6

1 medium head green or red cabbage cut into 3/4-inch wide ribbons
1/2 pound lentils
 3 garlic cloves, minced
6 ounces red potatoes, sliced 1/2 inch thick
1 medium onion, half chopped, half sliced
1 dried red chile
1 bay leaf
1 tablespoon chopped flat-leaf parsley
6 tbsp vegetable stock
3 1/2 cups water (or to taste)

Heat 4 tbsp vegetable stock in a large saucepan, medium heat. Add chopped half
of onion and cook, stirring often, until tender. Add 2 minced garlic cloves and
cook for less than a minute. Add lentils, water, chile, bay leaf, and bring to a
simmer. Reduce the heat, cover and simmer over low heat for 15 minutes. Add
potatoes. Continue to simmer for 30 minutes, or until the lentils and potatoes are
tender. While the lentils are simmering, cook cabbage with the remaining onion
and garlic in a skillet. Heat 2 tbsp vegetable stock over medium heat and add the
sliced onion for five minutes. Add one tbsp garlic and stir together for one
minute. Add cabbage and cook until the cabbage begins to wilt. Add 1/4 cup
water, turn the heat down to medium, cover and simmer 10 minutes, or until the
cabbage is tender and sweet, stirring from time to time. Spread cabbage over the
bottom of the pan in an even layer. Top with the lentils and potatoes. Sprinkle on
the parsley, and serve in wide soup bowls.

Soup – Minestrone
Makes about 2 1/2 quarts

2 cups dry kidney beans (*See Rules for Meal Preparation, Bean Preparation*)
 1 small onion, chopped
1 carrot, cut into chunks
1 celery stalk, sliced including top
1 potato, scrubbed and cut into chunks
1 small zucchini, diced
4 garlic cloves, minced
2 cups tomato juice
2 cups water or vegetable broth
1 cup finely chopped kale, collard greens, or spinach
2 tbsp chopped parsley
1/4 tsp black pepper
1/4 cup pasta shells
1 tbsp chopped fresh basil or 1 tsp dried basil
1 tsp mixed Italian herbs

Combine onion, garlic, carrot, celery, potato, and parsley in a large pot. Add tomato juice, water or broth, Italian herbs, and black pepper. Bring to a simmer, then cover and cook 20 minutes. Add zucchini, pasta, kidney beans, chopped greens, and basil. Cover and simmer until pasta is tender, about 20 minutes. Add extra tomato juice or water for a thinner soup.

Soup – Mushroom and Barley
Makes about 3 cups

2 cups water
1 cup cooked barley
1 4-ounce can mushrooms, including the liquid
2 tbsp barley flour
1/4 tsp garlic powder
pinch each of dried marjoram, sage, thyme, and dill weed

Place water and barley flour into blender. Blend on high speed for a few seconds. Add barley and blend until barley is chopped coarse. Add mushrooms with their liquid. Blend just enough to coarse-chop mushrooms. Transfer the blended mixture to a medium-sized saucepan and add all the remaining ingredients. Cook over medium heat until soup is hot and somewhat thickened.

Soup – Pumpkin

3 cups vegetable broth
15 oz. can pumpkin
1 cup chopped onion
1 garlic clove, crushed
1/2 tsp curry
1/4 tsp ground coriander
1/8 tsp cayenne pepper
1 cup water

Sauté onion and garlic in 2 tbsp water until soft but not browned. Add seasonings. Cook for one minute. Add broth and boil gently for 15-20 minutes. Stir in pumpkin and water. Cook for 5 minutes. Blend until creamy. Garnish with chives if desired.

Soup – Split Pea & Barley
Makes 8-9 cups

2 quarts water
1 carrot, chopped
3 stalks celery, diced
1 potato, diced
1 onion, diced
1 cup green split peas
1/4 cup barley
1 tsp celery seed
1/2 tsp basil
1/2 tsp thyme

Sauté onion and celery seed in a little water until onion is soft. Stir in peas and barley. Add water and bring to a boil. Cook on low heat, partially covered, for about an hour and a half. Add pepper, vegetable and herbs. Simmer another 30 to 45 minutes.

Soup – Tomato-Garlic

3 tbsp veggie broth or water
4 cloves garlic, pressed
1 tbsp paprika
8 cups tomato juice
1/2 cup nonalcoholic red wine (optional)

Sauté the garlic in the broth briefly, add paprika and let cook about a minute.
Add tomato juice and wine. Simmer for 5-10 minutes.

Soup – Vegetable Soup Raw
Serves 1

1/2 cup brown mushrooms, diced
1/2 cup zucchini, diced
1/2 cup carrot, diced
1/4 cup jicama, diced
1/4 cup celery, diced
1/2 cup sprouts
4 tbsp red onion, diced
1 tbsp herbs (e.g., parsley, thyme, oregano)
1 clove garlic, pressed
Pinch cayenne
Pinch ground black pepper
4 cups water

Place all ingredients in a bowl and stir well. Marinate in refrigerator for an hour.
Place half the stock in a blender and blend, then add it back to soup bowl. Mix
and serve.

Soup – Vegetable Soup with Hominy
Serves 4

1 15-ounce can of white hominy
1 1/2 cups stewed tomatoes with garlic, green pepper, and celery
4 carrots, sliced
3 cloves garlic, minced
1 large onion, chopped
1 red pepper, chopped
3 cups of water or low-sodium vegetable stock
1 cup green beans, broken into bite-sized lengths
3/4 tsp chili powder
1/2 tsp cumin
1/4 tsp pepper

In medium stock pot, braise garlic and onion in 1/2 cup water until soft. Add carrots and water or stock, and simmer 5 to 10 minutes. Drain and rinse hominy and add to the pot. Stir in the tomatoes, red pepper, green beans, and spices. Simmer for 15 minutes. Serve piping hot with little bowls of the toppings. Use salsa or chopped lettuce as toppings.

Stew – Green Split Pea and Barley

3 garlic cloves
2 large white potatoes, coarsely chopped
2 stalks celery, diced
2 large carrots, diced
6 cups water
2 cups chopped fresh spinach
1 medium yellow onion -- diced
1 cup green split peas -- rinsed
1/2 cup pearl barley
2 tbsp dried parsley
2 tbsp vegetable broth
2 tsp dried oregano or thyme leaves
1/2 tsp black pepper

In a large saucepan, heat the broth over medium heat. Add the onion, celery, carrots, and garlic and cook, stirring, for about 7 minutes. Add the water, split peas, barley, potatoes, parsley, oregano, and pepper and bring to a simmer over medium-high heat. Reduce the heat to medium and cook until peas are tender, about 1 hour. Stir in the spinach and cook over low heat for 10 to 15 minutes. Ladle into bowls and serve with warm whole wheat bread. (Note: To speed up the cooking time, soak the split peas in water for 1 hour before cooking.)

Stew – Lentil and Barley Stew
Makes about 1 1/2 quarts

1 small onion, chopped
1 garlic clove, pressed or minced
1 carrot, diced
1 celery stalk, sliced
1 quart vegetable broth or water
1/2 cup lentils, rinsed
1/4 cup hulled or pearled barley
1/2 tsp oregano
1/2 tsp ground cumin
1/4 tsp red pepper flakes
1/4 tsp black pepper

Place all ingredients into a large pot and bring to a simmer. Cover and cook, stirring occasionally, until lentils and barley are tender, about 1 hour.

Stew – Spicy Pumpkin
Serves 6

2 cups dry red kidney or pinto beans (*See Rules for Meal Preparation, Bean Preparation*)
1 cup fresh or frozen corn kernels
1 medium onion, thinly sliced
3-4 cups of small chunk (1/2-inch) raw pumpkin or butternut squash
1 cup vegetable stock
1 cup tomato sauce
1/2 cup salsa
1 tsp minced garlic
1 tsp chili powder
1/2 tsp hot red pepper flakes
1/2 tsp cumin
3-4 drops of Tabasco

Simmer pumpkin or squash in vegetable stock until tender. Add remaining ingredients and simmer uncovered over low heat for 30 minutes. Season to taste.

Stew – Summer
Makes about 2 1/2 quarts

2 cups dry cannelini beans or navy beans (*See Rules for Meal Preparation, Bean Preparation*)
1 12-ounce jar water-packed roasted red peppers, including liquid
5 large garlic cloves, minced
2 onions, chopped
4 cups eggplant, cut into 1/4-inch thick slices
3 cups zucchini, sliced
2 cups chopped fresh basil
1 green bell pepper, diced
1 cup water or vegetable broth
2 tbsp vegetable broth
1/4 tsp black pepper

Heat broth in a large pot, add onions. Cook over medium heat until onions are lightly browned. Add a small amounts of water if onions begin to stick. Add eggplant, bell pepper, and garlic, then cover and cook five minutes.. Coarsely chop red peppers and add, with their liquid. Add zucchini, basil, and water. Cover and cook over medium heat, stirring occasionally, for 3 minutes. Stir in cannelini beans and black pepper. Cover and cook until zucchini is just tender, about 3 minutes.

Mix-Ins/Side Dishes

Asparagus With Garlic & Pecans
Serves 4

1 pound asparagus, broken into bite-sized pieces
3 cloves garlic, minced
1/2 cup pecans, halved
1 tbsp low-sodium Tamari
2 tsp vegetable broth

Sauté garlic in broth in medium skillet. Add asparagus and Tamari. Cook 4-6 minutes stirring often until asparagus is tender. Add pecans, continue heating for 1-2 minutes and serve.

Asparagus With Raspberry Sauce
Serves 4

1 pound of asparagus
1 cup frozen raspberries
1/2 fresh orange or 1 tsp frozen orange juice concentrate
1 tsp orange zest (optional)

Put frozen raspberries in saucepot with orange juice or juice concentrate. Simmer until raspberries have fallen apart and mixture looks like a sauce. Remove from heat and set aside. Steam asparagus over hot water until just tender.. Pour sauce over asparagus. Serve hot or at room temperature. Garnish with orange zest, if desired.

Beans – Baked Beans
Makes about 8 cups

2-1/2 cups dry navy beans (or other small white beans) (*See Rules for Meal Preparation, Bean Preparation*)
1 cup tomato sauce
1 onion, chopped
1/2 cup molasses
2 tbsp vinegar
2 tsp stone ground or Dijon mustard
1 tsp Bakkon yeast (optional – found at health food stores)
1/2 tsp garlic granules or powder

Place beans in a large pot with onion. Add tomato sauce, molasses, mustard, vinegar, garlic granules and Bakkon yeast if using. Cook, loosely covered, over very low heat for 1 to 2 hours. Or, transfer to an ovenproof dish and bake at 350 for 2 to 3 hours.

Beans – Barbecued
Makes 6 cups

(*See Rules for Meal Preparation, Bean Preparation*)
2 cups dry pinto beans
2 cups dry kidney beans
1 10-ounce package frozen baby lima beans
1/2 cup crushed tomatoes
1 cup finely chopped onion
1 tbsp cider vinegar
1 tbsp molasses
2 tsp stone-ground mustard
1 tsp chili powder

Combine all ingredients in a saucepan and cook at a slow simmer for 25 to 30 minutes.

Beans – Black Beans and Tomatoes
Makes 4 cups

4 cups dry black beans (*See Rules for Meal Preparation, Bean Preparation*)
4 cups diced tomatoes
2 garlic cloves, minced
1/2 cup chopped onion
1/4 cup vegetable broth
2 tbsp canned, chopped green chilies
1 tbsp chopped cilantro or parsley
1/2 tsp cumin
1/2 tsp ground red pepper
1/4 tsp chili powder

Heat 1/4-cup vegetable broth in cooking skillet and heat over medium-high heat.
Add chopped onion and garlic. Sauté in broth until tender. Add tomatoes and
chilies. Reduce heat and cook uncovered 6 to 8 minutes or until mixture is
slightly thickened, stirring occasionally. Stir in beans and remaining ingredients.
Cover and cook five minutes or until thoroughly heated.

Beans – Refried Beans (spicy)
Makes about 5 cups

1 1/2 cups dry pinto beans
1 4-ounce can diced green chilies
4 garlic cloves, minced or pressed
1 onion, chopped
1 cup crushed or finely chopped tomatoes
1 1/2 tsp cumin
1/4 tsp cayenne

Clean and rinse beans, then soak in about 6 cups of water for 6 to 8 hours.
Discard soaking water, rinse beans and place in a large pot with 4 cups fresh
water, minced garlic, cumin, and cayenne. Simmer until tender, about 1 hour.
Heat 1/2 cup of water in a large skillet. Add onion and cook until soft, about 5
minutes. Stir in tomatoes and diced chilies. Cook, uncovered, over medium heat
for 10 minutes, stirring occasionally. Add cooked beans, including some cooking
liquid, a cup at a time to tomato mixture. Mash some of the beans as you add
them. When all the beans have been added, stir to mix, then cook over low heat,
stirring frequently, until thickened.

Beets in Dill Sauce
Makes about 4 cups

4 medium-sized beets
2 tbsp lemon juice
1 tbsp stone-ground mustard
1 tbsp cider vinegar
1 tbsp apple juice concentrate
1 tsp dried dill weed, or 1 tbsp fresh dill, chopped

Wash and peel the beets, then slice them into 1/4-inch thick rounds. Steam over boiling water until tender when pierced with a fork, about 20 minutes. Mix the remaining ingredients in a serving bowl. Add the beets and toss to mix. Serve immediately, or chill before serving.

Barley Cakes – Spinach
Makes 10 barley cakes

1 10-ounce package frozen spinach
1 small onion
2 medium garlic cloves
1 small carrot
2 cups fresh mushrooms
2 cups cooked barley
4 tbsp vegetable broth
2 tbsp shelled sunflower seeds

Grind the sunflower seeds in a food processor. Add the onion, garlic, carrot, and mushrooms. Grind thoroughly and then add the remaining ingredients and process for about 1 minute, or until well mixed. Preheat a large, skillet. Form the barley mixture into patties. Cook each side over medium-high heat for about 3 minutes, or until golden brown.

Broccoli and Ginger (sautéed)
Serves 4

1 clove garlic, minced
1 medium leek, sliced thin (white part only)
1/2-inch piece fresh ginger root, peeled and grated
1 pound broccoli, cut into florets
2 tbsp vegetable stock
4 tsp vegetable broth
1 tsp low-sodium Tamari

Sauté the garlic and ginger in the broth in a large skillet for 1 minute. Add the broccoli, leek, and stock. Toss together all the ingredients to mix well. Cover the pan and cook for 3 minutes. Remove the cover and continue to sauté, stirring frequently, until the vegetables are just tender, about 10 minutes.

Broccoli Slaw
Serves 6 - 8

4 broccoli stems, washed and peeled
6-inch long piece of daikon radish, peeled
2 kiwis, peeled and diced
2 large carrots, peeled
2 cloves garlic, minced
1/2 bunch green onions, chopped
2 tbsp pine nuts, toasted
1/4 tsp ground black pepper
2 tbsp water
Black sesame seeds

Coarsely grate broccoli stems, daikon radish, and carrots and put in a bowl. Add green onions, kiwis, pine nuts, garlic, salt, pepper, and water to bowl and toss together. Adjust seasoning to taste, and transfer to serving bowl. Garnish with black sesame seeds.

Bruschetta
Makes 1-1/2 cups

1 cup diced tomatoes, hearts discarded
2 garlic cloves, minced
1/4 cup diced red onion
1/4 cup minced fresh parsley
1/4 cup fresh basil, minced

Combine ingredients in glass or ceramic pan. Refrigerate until ready to serve. To serve, spoon onto thin slices of toasted whole wheat bread.

Buckwheat and Cabbage
Makes about 2½ cups

2 cups finely chopped cabbage
1 cup vegetable broth or water
1/2 cup buckwheat groats
4 tsp vegetable broth for sautéing

Heat broth in a large saucepan. Add kasha and shredded cabbage and cook over medium-high heat, stirring constantly, for 1 minute. Stir in 1 cup vegetable broth. Cover and simmer until buckwheat is tender and all the liquid is absorbed, about 10 minutes.

Collards or Kale – Braised
Makes 3 cups

1 bunch collard greens or kale (6 to 8 cups chopped)
2-3 garlic cloves, minced
1/4 cup water
2 tsp vegetable broth
2 tsp low-sodium Tamari (soy sauce)
1 tsp balsamic vinegar

Wash greens, remove stems, then chop leaves into 1/2-inch wide strips. Combine broth, Tamari, vinegar, garlic, and water in a large pot or skillet. Cook over high heat about 30 seconds. Reduce heat to medium-high, add chopped greens, and toss to mix. Cover and cook, stirring often, until greens are tender, about 5 minutes.

Cornbread
Serves 8

1-1/2 cups water
1 cup whole cornmeal
1 cup whole wheat pastry flour
4 tbsp vegetable broth
1-1/2 tbsp vinegar
2 tbsp maple syrup
1 tsp baking powder
1/2 tsp baking soda

Preheat oven to 425. Combine water and vinegar and let stand. Mix dry ingredients and maple syrup in a large bowl. Add the water mixture and the broth and stir until blended. Spread the batter into a 9-inch square baking dish and bake for 25 to 30 minutes or until done. Serve hot.

Crostini (herbed bread) with Roasted Red Peppers
Makes 1 baguette (about 20 slices)

10 sun-dried tomato halves
1 garlic clove, pressed
1 small whole wheat baguette, cut into 1/2-inch thick slices
1 cup boiling water
2/3 cup roasted red peppers (about 2 peppers)
2 tbsp fresh basil, finely chopped OR
1 tsp dried basil
1/8 tsp black pepper

Pour boiling water over tomatoes and set aside until softened, about 10 minutes.
Drain and chop coarsely. Chop roasted red peppers and add to tomatoes, along
with garlic, basil, and black pepper. Let stand 30 minutes. Preheat oven to 350.
Slice baguette and arrange slices in a single layer on one or two baking sheets.
Toast in preheated oven until outsides are crisp, 10 to 15 minutes. Remove from
oven and cool slightly, then spread each piece with 1 to 2 tablespoons of tomato
mixture.

Curried – Cauliflower with Peas (spicy)
Makes about 6 cups

1 10-ounce bag frozen peas
1 large onion, chopped
1 cauliflower, cut or broken into florets (about 4 cups)
1/2 cup vegetable broth or water
1-2 tbsp low-sodium Tamari (soy sauce)
1 tsp coriander
1 tsp whole mustard seed
1/2 tsp each: turmeric, cumin
1/4 tsp each: cinnamon, ginger, cardamom, cayenne pepper

Combine coriander, mustard seed, turmeric, cumin, cinnamon, ginger,
cardamom, and cayenne in a large skillet. Heat, stirring constantly, until spices
darken slightly and just begin to smoke: about one minute. Remove from heat
and cool slightly. Add vegetable broth, Tamari, and onion. Cook until onion is
soft, stirring occasionally, about five minutes. Stir in cauliflower, then cover and
cook over medium heat until tender when pierced with a fork, about five minutes.
Stir in peas and cook until hot, another minute or two. For a less spicy taste, cut
back on the cayenne pepper. Carrots and potatoes are optional.

Curried – Chickpea
Makes 8 to 10 servings

2 cups tomato sauce
4 cans of chickpeas, drained
8 cloves garlic, minced
2 1/2 medium onions, thinly sliced
2 green peppers, cut into small pieces
1/8 cup vegetable broth
2 tsp turmeric
1 tsp cumin
1 tsp allspice
1 1/2 tsp cayenne pepper
1/2 tsp ginger

Sauté the onions in the broth. When brown, add the tomato sauce, garlic and the spices and sauté for a few minutes. Add the chickpeas and the green peppers and sauté over fairly high heat until everything is browned, about 15 minutes. Add water, if needed, turn down the heat and cover. Simmer for about 1 hour, stirring frequently. Serve over rice.

Curried – Vegetables

1 1/2 cups tomatoes, diced
4 cardamoms, bruised
2 medium zucchinis, cut into 1 inch chunks
2 bay leaves
1 small onion, peeled and finely chopped
1 large potato, peeled and diced
1 small cauliflower, stalks removed and florets divided up
1/2 cup green beans
1/4 pint hot water
1 tbsp vegetable broth
1 tbsp turmeric
1 tsp fenugreek seeds
1 tsp coriander seeds
1/2 tsp mustard seeds
1/4 tsp freshly milled black pepper

Put onion into a very large bowl with broth and sautee until onions start to brown. Add the cardamoms, fenugreek, mustard, coriander seeds and turmeric and stir occasionally. Add the diced potato to the mixture until almost cooked. Add the zucchinis, cauliflower florets, beans, tomatoes and bay leaves and add about half the water. Reduce heat and cook until the vegetables are tender, adding the remaining water if necessary. Adjust seasoning to taste.

Garlic Bread
Makes about 20 slices

2 roasted garlic heads
1 loaf whole wheat French (or other) bread, sliced
1–2 tsp mixed Italian herbs

Preheat oven to 350. Peel roasted cloves or squeeze flesh from skin and place in a bowl. Mash with a fork, then mix in Italian herbs. Spread on sliced bread. Wrap tightly in foil and bake for 20 minutes.

Green Beans – Italian Style
Makes about 6 cups

1 pound fresh green beans
2 cups chopped tomatoes
2 large garlic cloves, minced
1 tbsp vegetable broth
2 tbsp chopped fresh basil or 1 tsp dried basil

Trim ends off beans and cut or break into bite-sized lengths. Steam until just tender, about 10 minutes, then set aside. Heat vegetable broth in a large skillet, then add tomatoes and garlic. Simmer 10 minutes. Add green beans and basil. Cook until beans are very tender, about 5 minutes, stirring occasionally. Season to taste.

Green Beans with Basil
Serves 4

1 lb. fresh or frozen green beans
1 tbsp minced onion
1 tsp vegetable broth
1 tsp dried basil leaves
1 tsp garlic powder
Dash pepper

Trim and snap green beans into thirds. Mince the onion. Put water on to boil to steam beans for 12-17 minutes or until tender. Sauté the onions in vegetable broth until tender. Add steamed beans, basil, garlic powder and pepper. Toss beans with basil sauce to coat evenly and serve.

Kale Crisps

1 bunch kale
2 tsp water
1 tsp red wine vinegar
Blackstrap molasses
Cayenne pepper to taste (optional)

Slice the hard vein out of the Kale. Chop into 2-3 inch strips. Wash and spin dry. In a mixing bowl toss the kale by hand with water and vinegar. Spread out on two parchment lined baking sheets. Bake at 350 degrees until crisp to the touch or about 10 minutes. Sprinkle molasses and cayenne pepper over strips.

Lentil – Bulgur Pilaf
6 servings

1 medium onion, minced
2 1/2 cups water
1 cup lentils
1 cup uncooked bulgur
1/2 cup minced fresh parsley
3 tbsp vegetable broth
1/2 tsp ground cumin
1/8 tsp cayenne pepper

Place lentils in a large saucepan. Add water and bring to a boil. Reduce heat, cover, and simmer for 15 minutes. Remove from heat. Stir in bulgur, cover, and set aside for 20 minutes, until bulgur is tender. Drain excess liquid. Heat broth in a skillet over medium heat. Add onion and sauté until lightly golden. Combine lentil-bulgur mixture, onion, parsley, cayenne pepper, and cumin in a large bowl and mix well.

Lentils – French Green
Makes about 6 cups

1 large onion, chopped
4 cups vegetable broth
1 cup French green lentils
1/2 cup chopped cilantro
1 tsp black mustard seeds
1 tsp turmeric
1 tsp cumin
1 tsp coriander
1/2 tsp ginger
1/4 tsp cayenne

Rinse lentils and place in a large pot with vegetable broth, onion and cilantro. Combine mustard seeds, turmeric, cumin, coriander, ginger, and cayenne in a small skillet. Toast over medium-high heat, stirring constantly, until spices are fragrant and just begin to smoke, about 2 minutes. Add to lentils. Cover and simmer until lentils are tender, about 30 minutes.

Mushrooms – In Barbeque Sauce
Serves 4

1 12-ounce package button or cremini mushrooms, sliced
1 small yellow onion, finely chopped
1/2 cup barbeque sauce

Braise onions in 1/4-cup water for 3-4 minutes. Add mushrooms and continue cooking for 4-5 more minutes. Add barbeque sauce and cook until sauce is desired thickness. Serve over veggie burgers, potatoes, or rice.

Polenta (cornmeal)
Makes 4 cups

4 cups water
1 cup polenta or stone-ground yellow cornmeal
1/2 tsp crushed dried rosemary (optional)

Bring water to a boil, then slowly pour in the polenta, stirring constantly with a whisk to prevent it from lumping. Lower heat and simmer, stirring fairly constantly until thick, about 10 minutes. (Note: polenta can be purchased at health food stores already prepared.)

Succotash

4 cups dry lima or kidney beans (*See Rules for Meal Preparation, Bean Preparation*)
2 cups whole-kernel corn
1 1/2 cups water
1/2 cup combination of red and green peppers, chopped

Combine all the ingredients in a large saucepan in water or a vegetable broth. Cook over low to medium heat, stirring the vegetables. Add the optional chopped sweet red and green pepper. Serves 4 to 6.

Sweet Potato Fries

4 large sweet potatoes cut like fries
2 tbsp maple syrup
1 tsp vegetable broth
1 tsp ground cinnamon

Toss cut vegetables, broth, cinnamon in a bowl. Transfer to baking sheet. Bake in a 450 oven for about 50 minutes, or until the vegetables are tender. During the last 30 minutes of roasting, toss vegetables occasionally. At the end of baking, toss with maple syrup.

Vegetable Korma

14 fl oz can coconut milk
2 oz flaked almonds
1 lb mixed vegetables cut into bite size chunks (e.g., carrot, potato, broccoli, cauliflower, peas)
1 onion, finely chopped
1 tbsp vegetable broth
1 tbsp curry paste

Heat the broth in a large saucepan and cook the onion over a fairly high heat for 5 minutes until golden brown. Stir in the curry paste and cook for 1 minute. Add the vegetables and coconut milk, cover and simmer for 15 minutes until the vegetables are tender. Place the almonds in a frying pan and dry fry for 2-3 minutes, tossing the almonds until golden brown. Season curry to taste with pepper and sprinkle over the toasted almonds. Serve immediately with rice, naan or bread.

Vegetables with Thai Peanut Sauce
Serves 5 to 8

Thai Peanut Sauce
4 cups vegetables, fruits, and nuts
2 tbsp vegetable broth
1 tbsp water
1 tbsp minced garlic

Use any combination of broccoli, carrots, cauliflower, red cabbage, green peppers, scallions, tomatoes, mushrooms, unsalted cashew halves, cilantro, raisins, and pineapple chunks totaling 4 cups. Sauté the vegetable/fruit/nut mixture with the water, garlic, and vegetable broth. Serve over rice topped with Peanut Sauce.

Dinner

Basmati, Vegetables & Fruit
Serves 4

3 cups pineapple chunks
2 unripe bananas
1 medium onion, cubed
1 medium carrot, grated
2 cups broccoli florets
1 cup basmati rice
2 tbsp vegetable broth
1 tbsp chopped parsley
1 tbsp chopped chives
1 tbsp chopped fresh basil
1/2 tsp curry powder

Cook the rice in 2 cups of water for 20 minutes, or until done. Cut the broccoli florets into small flowers. Cut the pineapple into bite-sized pieces and the banana into large slices. Heat the broth in a pan, and add the onion. Add the broccoli and carrot. Lower the heat, cover the pan and let it simmer for a few minutes. Add the curry, pineapple, banana and pepper, and fry for a few more minutes. The vegetables should be just tender. Add the herbs shortly before serving. Serve on rice.

Basmati and Wild Rice Pilaf
Makes about 6 cups

2 garlic cloves, minced
2 stalks celery, thinly sliced
1 onion, finely chopped
2-1/2 cups vegetable broth
2 cups thinly sliced mushrooms
1/2 cup wild rice, rinsed
1/2 cup brown basmati rice, rinsed
1/3 cup chopped pecans
1/3 cup finely chopped parsley
1/2 tsp thyme
1/2 tsp marjoram
1/4 tsp black pepper

Combine wild rice and vegetable broth in a saucepan. Cover and simmer 20 minutes. Add basmati rice, then cover and continue cooking over very low heat until tender, about 50 minutes. Preheat oven to 375. Place pecans in a small oven-proof dish and bake until fragrant, about 8 minutes. Set aside. Heat 1/2 cup of water in a large skillet and cook onion and garlic until all the water has evaporated. Add 1/4 cup of water and cook until the water has evaporated. Repeat until onions are browned, about 20 minutes. Lower heat slightly and add mushrooms, celery, parsley, thyme, marjoram and black pepper. Cook, stirring frequently, for 5 minutes. Add cooked rice and toasted pecans. Stir to mix, then transfer to a baking dish and bake 20 minutes.

Broccoli with Buckwheat and Black Bean Sauce
Makes about 8 cups

2 cups dry black beans (*See Rules for Meal Preparation, Bean Preparation*)
1 large bunch broccoli
4 cups boiling water
2 cups buckwheat groats (or kasha for stronger flavor)
1/2 cup roasted red pepper
2 tbsp lemon juice
2 tbsp vegetable broth
1/2 tsp chili powder
1/4 tsp ground cumin
1/4 tsp ground coriander
1/4 cup chopped fresh cilantro

Cut off broccoli stems. Cut or break the tops into bite-sized florets. Peel the stem with a sharp knife, then slice into 1/2-inch thick rounds. Set aside. Into the water in a large saucepan, place buckwheat groats. Cover and simmer for about 10 minutes, or until all the liquid has been absorbed. While buckwheat (kasha) is cooking, combine and purée all the remaining ingredients in a food processor or blender. Just before you are ready to eat, steam broccoli over boiling water for about 5 minutes, or until it is bright green and just tender. Place a generous about of buckwheat on each serving plate, then top with steamed broccoli and black-bean sauce.

Buckwheat (roasted) Pilaf
Serves 4

1 small carrot, sliced
1 small onion, cut in 8 pieces
1/2 celery rib, sliced
2 cups vegetable broth
1/2 cup whole buckwheat groats (aka kasha)

In a food processor, pulse the carrot, onion and celery until they are finely chopped. In a large, heavy saucepan or small Dutch oven, heat the 2 tablespoons of broth over medium-high heat. Stir in the chopped vegetables. Sauté until they are soft, 4 minutes, stirring occasionally. Mix the buckwheat into the sautéed vegetables. Stir until it is fragrant and looks slightly darker in color, 1-2 minutes. Pour in the broth. Cover the pot tightly. When the liquid boils, reduce the heat and simmer 10 minutes. Turn off the heat and let the pilaf sit 5 minutes. Fluff the pilaf with a fork.

Bulgur Pilaf (spicy)
Makes about 4 cups

1 medium onion, chopped
2 garlic cloves, minced
1/2 red bell pepper, finely diced
1-3/4 cups boiling water or vegetable stock
1 cup bulgur wheat
2 tbsp vegetable broth
2 tsp chili powder
3/4 tsp cumin
1/8 tsp celery seed

Heat broth in a large skillet or pot and cook onion for 3 minutes. Stir in garlic, bulgur, chili powder, cumin, and celery seed. Continue cooking, stirring often, until onion is soft, about 5 minutes. Add bell pepper and boiling water. Stir to mix, then cover and simmer until bulgur is tender and all liquid is absorbed, about 20 minutes. Oven method: Preheat oven to 350. Prepare as above, except before adding boiling water, transfer bulgur mixture to an ovenproof dish. Add boiling water, cover with foil and bake until bulgur is tender and all liquid is absorbed, about 30 minutes.

Bulgur – Spanish
Serves 8

3-1/2 cups boiling water
2 cups bulgur
2 garlic cloves, minced
4-6 tsp chili powder
2 tsp vegetable broth
1 tsp ground cumin

Place the bulgur in a large bowl and pour the boiling water over it. Cover the bowl and let stand 20 minutes, until the bulgur is tender. Drain off any excess water. In a large skillet, sauté the garlic in vegetable broth (or water). Do not let it brown. With the pan still on the heat, stir in the soaked bulgur and add the chili powder and cumin. Turn with a spatula to mix in the spices and continue cooking until the mixture is very hot.

Burger – Beet
Serves 6

1 cup uncooked oats
1/2 cup cooked oats
1/2 cup coarsely ground walnuts
1/4 cup coarsely ground almonds
1/4 cup minced green pepper
1/4 cup minced onion
2 tbsp low-sodium Tamari (soy sauce)
2 tbsp sesame seeds
1 tbsp instant dry vegetable broth
1 tbsp nutritional yeast flakes (optional)
1 tbsp finely grated raw beet
1 tsp dried basil
1/4 tsp dried thyme
1/4 tsp ground sage
1/4 tsp mustard powder
tomato slices, for garnish

Mix all ingredients together well. Form into 6 patties and grill until cooked through. Serve on whole wheat rolls with tomato slices and your favorite condiments.

Burger – Lentil
Makes 8 burgers

1 small onion, chopped
1/2 cup short-grain brown rice
1/2 cup lentils
2 cups water
1 small carrot
1 medium-sized celery stalk
2 tsp stone-ground mustard
1 tsp garlic powder
Vegetable oil substitute, for skillet

In a medium-sized saucepan, combine onion, rice, lentils, and water. Bring to a slow simmer, then cover and cook for about 50 minutes, or until rice and lentils are tender and all the water has been absorbed. Chop carrot and celery until fine (a food processor makes this easy). Add them to the hot lentil mixture, along with the remaining ingredients. Stir to mix, then chill completely. (You can make the patties while the mixture is still warm, but forming is much easier once it is chilled.) Form mixture into 2- to 3-inch patties. Lightly coat a large skillet with a vegetable oil substitute (e.g., pureed bananas). Cook patties over medium heat for about 4 minutes per side, or until lightly browned.

Burger – Nut and Seed
Makes 4 burgers

1 carrot, grated
1 stalk celery, finely chopped
1/2 cup ground almonds
1/2 cup ground raw sunflower seeds
1/2 cup finely chopped onion
1 tbsp vegetable broth
1 tsp dill weed
1 tsp marjoram
Egg replacer equivalent to 1 egg
Garlic powder to taste
Black pepper to taste

Preheat oven to 350. Grind the nuts in a coffee grinder or food processor, and chop vegetables into small pieces. Mix all the ingredients together, and shape into burgers. Bake for 15 minutes on each side on a cookie sheet.

Chili – Black Bean
Makes 6 cups

4 cups dry black beans (*See Rules for Meal Preparation, Bean Preparation*)
1 4-ounce can diced chilies
2 medium-sized cloves garlic, minced
1 medium-sized onion, chopped
1 small bell pepper, diced fine
1/2 cup water
1/2 cup crushed tomatoes or tomato sauce
1 tsp ground cumin

In a large skillet or pot, heat the water. Add onion, garlic, and pepper. Cook over high heat until onion is translucent. Add remaining ingredients and simmer for about 15 minutes or until flavors are blended.

Chili – Three Bean

(*See Rules for Meal Preparation, Bean Preparation*)
4 cups tomatoes, diced
2 cups dry white beans
2 cups dry black beans
2 cups dry red beans
1 1/2 cup tomato sauce
1 1/2 cups chopped onion
2 tbsp maple syrup
2 tbsp minced garlic
1 tbsp chili powder
2 tsp ground cumin
2 tsp vegetable broth
1 tsp black pepper

Heat broth in large pot over medium-high heat. Cook onions until soft. Drain and rinse three beans and add to onions. Stir in all remaining ingredients. Bring to a boil and then reduce heat to low and simmer for 30 to 45 minutes.

Chili – Vegetarian
Serves 4

4 cups dry pinto beans (*See Rules for Meal Preparation, Bean Preparation*)
 1-3 jalapeno peppers, seeded and minced
1 medium yellow onion, chopped
1 medium green bell pepper, cut in ½-inch pieces
1 cup coarsely chopped tomatoes
2 cups vegetable broth, divided
1/4 cup chopped cilantro leaves
2 tsp ground ancho chile, or 1 Tbs. chili powder
1 tbsp finely chopped garlic
1 tsp ground cumin
1 tsp dried oregano
2 tsp masa or corn meal
Freshly ground black pepper, optional

In a medium Dutch oven, sauté the onion, bell pepper and garlic in a small amount of vegetable broth until the onion is translucent.. Add the jalapeno pepper, cumin, ancho chile or chili powder and oregano. Stir until the spices are fragrant. Add the beans, chopped tomatoes, all but 3 tablespoons of the vegetable broth and the cilantro. Set the remaining vegetable broth aside. Bring the chili to a boil. Reduce the heat and simmer, uncovered, for 10 minutes. Place the masa or corn meal in a small bowl. Mix in the reserved vegetable broth, stirring to make a smooth mixture. While stirring the chili, blend in the corn mixture, blending it in well. Add pepper, if desired. Continue simmering the chili 10 minutes longer. For the best flavor, let the chili sit 1-2 hours in the refrigerator. Reheat and serve.

Couscous – Moroccan
Serves 4

1 15-oz. can chick peas
1 sweet potato or small winter squash, cubed
1 zucchini, cubed
1 red bell pepper, diced
1 yellow bell pepper, diced
1 clove garlic, minced or pressed
2 cups uncooked couscous
1/2 cup raisins
1/4 cup water
2 tbsp vegetable broth
1 tsp ground cumin
1/2 tsp allspice
1/2 tsp ground ginger
1/2 tsp turmeric
1/2 tsp paprika
1/4 tsp cayenne
1/4 tsp cinnamon

Sauté the zucchini, sweet potato or squash, and garlic in the broth until partially cooked, about 5 minutes. Use water as necessary to keep the vegetables from sticking. Drain and rinse the chick peas. Add the spices, chick peas, and pepper to the pan. Cover and cook for about 5 minutes. Meanwhile, place the couscous and raisins in another saucepan. Add enough water so that the couscous is covered by about 1/2 inch. Bring the mixture to a boil, then cover tightly, remove from the heat, and let set for at least 10 minutes. Remove the cover from the pepper/chick pea mixture, stir, and cook a few minutes longer to heat thoroughly and thicken.

Curried – Mushrooms, Avocados & Rice

Cooked rice
4 avocadoes
2 tomatoes
1 lb mushrooms
1 large onion
2 tbsp vegetable broth
2 tsp (or more to taste) curry powder
4 tsp lemon juice

Chop the onion. Sauté in the broth along with the mushrooms until tender. Stir in the curry powder and cook for a few moments longer. Chop the tomato and add to the saucepan. Heat through. Add the lemon juice. Stir well and heat until just below boiling point. Peel and halve the avocados. Place on the rice and fill with the mushroom mixture.

Eggplant "Steaks"
Makes 4 servings

2 small eggplants
1 clove garlic, minced
1 tbsp balsamic vinegar
6 tbsp vegetable broth
1 tsp minced fresh parsley
1/2 tsp hot sauce
1/3 tsp dried rosemary

Remove the stem ends from the eggplants and cut off enough of the skin to square the sides. Slice each eggplant lengthwise into two pieces, each approximately 1/2-inch thick. Heat the oven to 350. In a small bowl, stir together 2 tablespoons of broth and the hot sauce. Brush evenly over both sides of the eggplant slices. Bake on a baking sheet for 15 minutes, turning over once. Then broil for 1 minute per side or until the slices are well browned and tender. In a small bowl, stir together the remaining broth, garlic, vinegar, parsley, and rosemary. Brush on the cooked eggplant. Let stand for 5 minutes before serving.

Falafel

2 15 oz cans chickpeas
6 scallions, minced
4 cloves garlic, minced
1/3 cup whole wheat flour (or brown rice flour, quinoa flour)
1/4 cup minced fresh parsley
1/4 cup water
1 tbsp lemon juice
1 tsp turmeric
cayenne to taste

Mix everything but flour in food processor (or mash it). Add flour and stir till well mixed. Form into small patties. Bake at 375, turn, until both sides are crispy. Wrap in spinach leaves. Dip in favorite dressing.

Ginger Noodles
Serves 6 to 8

1 package whole wheat soba noodles (approximately 8 ounces)
2 garlic cloves, minced
2 green onions, finely chopped, including tops
1/4 cup fresh cilantro (optional)
1 jalapeno pepper, finely chopped
3 tbsp seasoned rice vinegar
3 tbsp low-sodium Tamari (soy sauce)
2 tsp finely chopped fresh ginger

Cook the noodles in boiling water according to the package directions. When tender, drain, and rinse. Mix all the remaining ingredients, then pour over the noodles and toss to mix.

Greens and Beans With Garlic
Serves 4

2 cups dry cannellini beans (*See Rules for Meal Preparation, Bean Preparation*)
2 large cloves garlic, minced
3 cups chopped kale
3 cups chopped broccoli
2 cups collards, cut in 1/2-inch ribbons
3 cups fresh spinach or a 10 oz. frozen package, defrosted
1 cup vegetable broth
3/4 cup small leek, white part only, sliced
1/2 cup scallions, green and white parts, chopped
Season to taste.

In a large, heavy skillet over medium heat, sauté the leeks, scallions and garlic in a few tbsp of vegetable broth. Add the kale, broccoli rabe and collards, stirring until they are wilted. Mix in spinach and beans. Add the vegetable broth and simmer until the greens are tender, stirring occasionally. Season to taste. Serve over pasta or polenta.

Mushrooms – Portabello Grilled
Serves 4

4 large portabello mushrooms
2 medium-size cloves garlic, minced
4 tsp of vegetable broth
2 tbsp of red wine
2 tbsp low-sodium Tamari (soy sauce)
1 tbsp of balsamic vinegar

Clean mushrooms and trim stems flush with the bottom of the caps. In a large skillet, mix the remaining ingredients. Heat until the mixture begins to bubble; add mushrooms, tops down. Reduce to medium heat. Cover and cook for about 3 minutes, or until tops are browned. (If pan becomes dry, add 2 to 3 tbsp of water.) Turn the mushrooms and cook for about 5 minutes more, or until tender when pierced with a sharp knife.

Pasta – Artichoke
Makes 4 servings

1 (14-oz.) can artichoke hearts, quartered
2 cups tomatoes, diced
1 1/2 cups tomato sauce
1/2 pound tri-colored whole wheat pasta
2 cloves garlic, minced
1/2 medium onion, chopped
2 tbsp vegetable broth

Cook the pasta according to the package directions. While the pasta is cooking, sauté the onion and garlic in the broth for 1 to 2 minutes. Add the artichokes, tomatoes, and tomato sauce. Drain the pasta and combine all the ingredients.

Pasta – Asparagus
Serves 4

2 pounds fresh asparagus
2 1/2 cups tomatoes, chopped
8 ounces spaghetti
1 medium onion, chopped
2 tbsp water or vegetable stock
1 tbsp chopped fresh basil
1/4 tsp ground sage

Heat water or vegetable stock in a large, pan. Add onion and sauté over medium heat for 3 minutes, until translucent. Add tomatoes, asparagus, basil, and sage. Bring to a boil, cover, and simmer for 7 minutes. Remove from heat and keep warm. Cook pasta in water only without salt. Drain pasta and place in a serving bowl. Add the asparagus mixture and toss.

Pasta – Buckwheat Pasta
Serves 6

12 ounces whole wheat soba noodles
1 medium onion, chopped
3 cups sliced fresh mushrooms
1-1/2 cups cold water
4 tbsp vegetable broth
2 tbsp whole wheat flour
2 tsp low-sodium Tamari (soy sauce)
1/2 tsp garlic powder
1/4 tsp black pepper

Sauté the onion in a large skillet with the broth until transparent, then add the mushrooms. Cover and continue cooking until mushrooms are brown. Whisk flour and water together until smooth, then add to the skillet along with the Tamari, garlic powder, and pepper. Cook, uncovered, over medium-low heat until thickened. Bring water to boil in a large kettle. Add the noodles and boil until al dente, about 8 minutes.

Pasta – Cold Linguine & Asparagus
Makes 4 servings

3/4 lb. asparagus, cut diagonally into 1 1/2-inch pieces
8 oz. linguine whole wheat pasta
1/2 cup orange juice (unsweetened)
1/2 cup sliced green onions (green part only)
2 tbsp low-sodium Tamari (soy sauce)
3 tsp vegetable broth
1 tsp minced roasted garlic
1 tsp grated, fresh ginger root
1 tsp grated orange peel
1/4 tsp brown sugar
Dash hot pepper sauce, or to taste

Cook the noodles according to the package directions. Place the asparagus in a colander. Pour the noodles into the colander, on top of the asparagus, and drain—the hot water and noodles will lightly steam the asparagus. Leave in the colander for 10 minutes. Combine the remaining ingredients in a large bowl and mix well. Add the noodles and asparagus and stir gently until well blended. Refrigerate for several hours or overnight, stirring occasionally. Stir again before serving and serve cold.

Pasta – Lentils and Artichoke Hearts

1 pound farfalle, rotini or other whole wheat pasta
1 1/2 cups artichoke hearts
2 large garlic cloves, pressed or minced
1 bay leaf
1 cup dry red lentils
3 cups water
2 cups tomatoes, coarsely chopped
2 cups diced onions
2 tbsp lemon juice
2 tsp ground cumin
1 tsp ground coriander
1/4 tsp crushed red pepper

Combine the water, lentils, and bay leaf, bring to a boil, lower the heat and simmer for 15-20 min. Sauté onions until golden, add the garlic, cumin, and coriander, stir frequently. Add the lemon juice, tomatoes, artichoke hearts and crushed red pepper and simmer for 10 minutes. Drain the cooked lentils, save some of the cooking liquid (in case sauce is dry). Then add lentils to the tomato mixture, simmer for 10 minutes, adding 1/2 cup of the cooking liquid from lentils if sauce is dry. Boil water for pasta, and then top the pasta with the sauce.

Pasta – Mediterranean

12 or more kalamata olives
4 spring onions, sliced
2 sweet red peppers, sliced thinly
2 cloves of garlic, minced
3 tbsp vegetable broth
Fettuccini, linguini or angel hair

Over a medium flame, sauté the garlic in the broth for a minute. Add the green onions and sauté 2 more minutes. Add the olives and peppers and sauté a few more minutes then take it off heat and serve it over the pasta.

Pasta – Penne with Fresh Spinach, Tomatoes, and Olives
Serves 4

3 cups tomatoes, diced
8 ounces whole wheat penne pasta
1 pound fresh spinach, coarsely chopped
1 medium onion, chopped
1/2 cup kalamata olives, pitted, sliced
2 tbsp vegetable broth
1 tbsp chopped fresh parsley

Heat broth in a large skillet. Add onion and sauté over medium heat for 3 minutes. Add chopped tomatoes. Bring to a boil and then reduce heat, cover, and simmer for 20 minutes. Add sliced olives, chopped spinach, and parsley. Cook an additional 5 minutes. Meanwhile, cook pasta. Drain and transfer to a serving bowl. Add spinach mixture and toss.

Pasta – Roasted Vegetables
Serves 6

16-ounces penne or other bite-sized pasta
10-12 baby bella or cremini mushrooms, quartered
2 Roma tomatoes, chopped
1 medium zucchini, quartered and sliced
1 sweet red pepper, cut into bite-sized chunks
1 small onion, cut into bite-sized chunks
1/2 large eggplant, cut into bite-sized chunks
1/2 head garlic (about 6 cloves)
2 tbsp vegetable broth
2 tsp fresh thyme
crushed red pepper, to taste (optional)

Heat oven to 400. Peel garlic cloves and cut in half. Spread eggplant, zucchini, red pepper, onion, mushrooms, and garlic cloves on a flat pan (baking dish or cookie sheet). Sprinkle with 1 tablespoon of vegetable broth and toss. Roast for 25 to 35 minutes, turning vegetables once during cooking, until vegetables are soft and have crispy edges. Cook pasta according to package directions, drain, and rinse. Toss pasta with vegetables, tomatoes, fresh thyme, and the remaining tablespoon of broth. Serve warm or at room temperature.

Pasta Supper
Makes about 6 cups

2 cups red kidney beans (*See Rules for Meal Preparation, Bean Preparation*)
8 ounces whole wheat pasta spirals
1 onion chopped
2 cups finely chopped fresh kale
1 cup tomato juice
1/2 cup chopped fresh basil
1/4 cup chopped garlic
1 tbsp vegetable broth

Cook the pasta until just tender. Transfer to a colander. Rinse and drain. Set aside. Heat the broth in a large skillet or pot. Add the onion and garlic and cook over medium heat, stirring often. Stir in 1/4 cup of water. Add the tomato juice, kidney beans, kale and basil. Stir to mix, then cover and simmer until the kale is tender. Stir in the cooked pasta.

Penne with Kale, Tomatoes and Olives
Serves 4

2 1/2 cups tomatoes, diced
1 bunch kale, de-stemmed and diced
1 medium onion, chopped
1/2 cup kalamata olives, pitted and sliced
1/2 cup chopped fresh parsley
8 ounces whole-wheat penne pasta
½ cup water

Heat water in a large skillet. Add onion and sauté over medium heat for 3 minutes. Add diced tomatoes. Bring to a boil and then reduce heat, cover, and simmer for 20 minutes. Add sliced olives, chopped spinach or kale, and parsley. Cook an additional 5 minutes.
Meanwhile, cook pasta according to package directions. Drain and transfer to a serving bowl. Add tomato mixture and toss gently. Serve immediately.

Pie – Tamale

2 cups dry kidney beans (*See Rules for Meal Preparation, Bean Preparation*)
1 1/2 cups fresh or frozen corn kernels
1 can sliced or whole black olives
1 chopped onion
1 chopped bell pepper
1 1/2 pints tomatoes
1 cup cornmeal
1/2 cup water
1 tbsp chili powder
Garlic powder

Mix all together and pour into casserole. Bake at 350, covered, for 30 min. Uncover to brown top.

Pizza
Makes 4 servings.

4 individual whole wheat pizza shells
1 small eggplant, sliced
1 medium zucchini, sliced
1 red onion, cut into small wedges
1 red bell pepper, thinly sliced
1 yellow bell pepper, thinly sliced
2 tbsp vegetable broth
1 tbsp balsamic vinegar
1/2 tsp dried thyme
1/2 tsp black pepper
1/2 cup tomato sauce

Preheat the oven to 425. Combine the eggplant, zucchini, onion, bell peppers, broth, vinegar, thyme, and pepper in a large baking dish and toss to mix well. Bake, stirring occasionally, for 20 minutes, or until the vegetables are tender. Set aside. Place the pizza shells on baking sheets. Spread about 2 tablespoons of the tomato sauce on each pizza shell, then top with the roasted vegetables. Bake for 10 to 12 minutes or until the pizza shells and vegetables are heated through.

Pizza – Pita Pizzas
Makes 6 pizzas

6 pieces of whole wheat pita bread
1 1/2 cup tomato sauce
1 6-ounce can tomato paste
2 green onions, thinly sliced
1 red bell pepper, diced
1 cup chopped mushrooms
1 tsp garlic granules or powder
1/2 tsp basil
1/2 tsp oregano
1/2 tsp thyme

Preheat oven to 375. Combine tomato sauce, tomato paste, garlic granules and herbs. Prepare vegetables as directed. Turn a piece of pita bread upside down and spread with 2 to 3 tablespoons of sauce. Top with chopped vegetables. Repeat with remaining pita breads. Arrange on a baking sheet and bake until edges are lightly browned, about 10 minutes. (Note: Refrigerate or freeze the remaining sauce for use at another time or use with another meal.)

Polenta – Grilled with Portabella Mushrooms
Serves 4

4 large portabella mushrooms
1 roasted red pepper, cut into thin strips for garnish (optional)
2 cups vegetable broth
1/2 cup polenta (coarsely ground cornmeal)
1/2 cup water
2 tbsp vegetable broth
2 tbsp low-sodium Tamari (soy sauce)
2 tbsp balsamic vinegar
2 tbsp red wine
2 garlic cloves, crushed

Combine the polenta, 2 cups vegetable broth, and the 1/2 cup of water in a saucepan. Bring to a simmer and cook, stirring frequently, until very thick, 15 to 20 minutes. Pour into a 9- x 9-inch baking dish and chill completely. To grill, cut into wedges and cook over medium heat until nicely browned. Clean the mushrooms, remove stems. Prepare the marinade by stirring the remaining ingredients together in a large bowl. Place the mushrooms upside down in the marinade and let stand 10 to 15 minutes. Turn right side up and grill over medium-hot coals about 5 minutes. Turn and pour some of the marinade into each of the cavities. Grill until mushrooms can be pierced with a skewer, about 5 minutes longer. Serve with grilled polenta. Garnish with roasted red pepper strips, if desired.

Polenta – Stuffed Peppers
Makes 4 servings.

1 (1-lb.) package cooked polenta
2 medium tomatoes, diced
1 green, 1 red, 1 yellow, and 1 orange bell pepper (or any combination you choose)
2 tbsp vegetable broth
1/2 tsp minced fresh garlic
1/4 tsp pepper
Paprika

Preheat the oven to 375. Cut the tops off the peppers and scoop out the insides. Place peppers on a baking tray. Sauté the garlic in the broth over low heat. Add the tomatoes and pepper. Heat briefly and stir into the polenta.
Fill the peppers with the polenta mixture and sprinkle with paprika. Cook for 30 to 40 minutes.

Quesadillas
Makes 8 quesadillas

2 cups dry garbanzo beans (*See Rules for Meal Preparation, Bean Preparation*)
8 corn tortillas
1 garlic clove, peeled
1/2 cup chopped green onions
1/2 cup salsa
1/2 cup water-packed, roasted red pepper
3 tbsp lemon juice
1 tbsp vegetable broth
1/4 tsp cumin

Place garbanzo beans in a food processor or blender with roasted peppers, lemon juice, broth, garlic, and cumin. Process until very smooth, 1 to 2 minutes. Spread a tortilla with 2 to 3 tablespoons of garbanzo mixture and place in a large skillet over medium heat. Sprinkle with chopped green onions, and salsa. Top with a second tortilla and cook until the bottom tortilla is warm and soft, 2-3 minutes. Turn and cook the second side for another minute. Remove from pan and cut in half. Repeat with remaining tortillas.

Ratatouille
Makes 4 to 5 servings.

4-5 cloves garlic, crushed
2 large tomatoes, cut into medium wedges
1 medium zucchini, sliced
1 green bell pepper, chopped
1 red bell pepper, chopped
1 small eggplant, cut into small cubes
1 large onion, diced
1 bay leaf
1/2 cup tomato juice
5 tbsp tomato paste
4 tbsp dry red wine
1 tbsp vegetable broth
1 tbsp dried basil
1/2 tbsp dried marjoram
1/2 tbsp dried oregano
1/2 tsp black pepper
Dash of ground rosemary

Sauté the onion in the broth until translucent. Add the bay leaf and tomato juice and stir well. Then add the garlic, herbs and pepper and mix until well blended. Cover the saucepan and simmer for 10 minutes over low heat. Add the zucchini and peppers, stir well, cover, and simmer for another 5 minutes. Add the eggplant, tomatoes, and tomato paste and stir again. Cover and continue to simmer until the vegetables are tender, about 8 minutes more. Serve over rice or with crusty French bread.

Rotini with Ginger Peanut Sauce
Serves 6

8 ounces rotini
2 tbsp peanut butter
1 to 2 tbsp chopped fresh ginger root
1 tbsp low-sodium Tamari (soy sauce)
1-1/2 tbsp vinegar
1 tsp Dijon mustard
1 cup steamed carrots
1 cup steamed broccoli
3 scallions, finely chopped

Boil the rotini until tender. Drain, saving 1/2 cup of the water. In a blender, whir the 1/2-cup pasta water and the ginger, peanut butter, Tamari, vinegar, and mustard. Toss pasta with sauce. Top with carrots, broccoli, and chopped scallions. (Note: you can use prepared peanut sauce instead of making it.)

Sandwich – Chickpea Pita Pockets

4 whole wheat pitas
1 16 oz can chick peas, rinsed, drained and mashed
1/3 cup chopped celery
1 tsp minced onion
2 tsp pickle relish (or piccalilly)
2 tsp mustard
Dash of garlic powder
Lettuce, tomato slices, grated carrot, etc for toppings

Place the chickpeas, celery, onion, relish, mustard and garlic powder in a bowl and mix well. Cut the pitas in half and open up into pockets. Fill each pita pocket with 1/4 of the chickpea spread, top with lettuce, tomato or other vegetables and serve.

Sandwich – Garbanzo Salad
Makes 4 sandwiches

2 cups dry garbanzo beans (*See Rules for Meal Preparation, Bean Preparation*)
8 slices whole wheat bread
4 lettuce leaves
4 tomato slices
1 stalk celery, finely sliced
1 green onion, finely chopped
1 tbsp sweet pickle relish

Mash garbanzo beans with a fork or potato masher, leaving some chunks. Add sliced celery, chopped onion and pickle relish. Spread on whole wheat bread and top with lettuce and sliced tomatoes.

Sandwich – Grilled Portobello
Serves 4

4 large Portobello mushrooms
4 whole wheat buns
1 cup red wine vinegar
1 cup vegetable broth
1 cup low-sodium Tamari (soy sauce)
Grilled onion

Take equal parts of red wine vinegar, vegetable broth and Tamari and place in a blender to mix then pour over the mushrooms. Let them sit overnight then grill. Add onion and other toppings and a bun.

Sandwich – Toasted Wheat Roll

Whole wheat sandwich roll
Lettuce
Tomato
Onions
Pickles
Pepperoncini (Tuscan peppers)
Basil
Pepper
Dijon Mustard
Slice ingredients so they all fit onto a sandwich roll. Toast bun. Add mustard and any other seasoning or sauce.

Spinach with Garlic
Serves 4

1 large bunch of fresh spinach
3 cloves of garlic
1 tsp vegetarian Worcestershire sauce

Wash and de-stem spinach. Peel and mince garlic. Braise garlic in Worcestershire sauce over medium heat, stirring, until lightly browned. Add spinach to hot skillet. Use tongs to turn spinach until it is just wilted. Serve hot or at room temperature.

Squash – Pinto Beans
Makes 4 servings

2 cups dry pinto beans (*See Rules for Meal Preparation, Bean Preparation*)
1 cup diced tomatoes
2 garlic cloves, minced
3 thyme sprigs
2 cups hot cooked brown rice
1 cup (1/2-inch-thick) sliced yellow squash
1 cup (1/2-inch-thick) sliced zucchini
1/2 cup fresh corn kernels
1/2 cup chopped onion
1/4 cup vegetable broth (or more, as needed, to sauté in)
2 tsp minced seeded jalapeno pepper

Heat broth in a large skillet over medium-high heat. Add the onion, jalapeno, and garlic, and sauté 2 minutes. Stir in squash and zucchini, and sauté 2 minutes. Add corn, beans, tomatoes, and thyme; cover, reduce heat, and simmer 10 minutes. Discard thyme. Serve over rice.

Squash – Spanish
Serves 4

1 8-ounce package of button mushrooms, sliced
2 small zucchini, quartered lengthwise and sliced
1 small yellow onion, finely chopped
1-1/2 cups frozen corn
2 tbsp water
1/2 tsp cumin
1/2 tsp chili powder

Braise onion in 1 tablespoon of water, stirring until liquid has evaporated. Add sliced zucchini, mushrooms, and the remaining water. Stir in spices and simmer for 5 minutes, covered, until mushrooms are soft. Stir in corn and cook for 2 more minutes to heat through. Add black pepper to taste.

Squash – Winter
Makes 4 cups

1 medium winter squash (e.g., butternut)
1/2 cup water
2 tsp low-sodium Tamari (soy sauce)
2 tbsp maple syrup

Slice the squash in half and then peel and remove the seeds. Cut the squash into 1-inch cubes. Place cubes into a large pot with the water. Add the Tamari and syrup. Cover and simmer over medium heat for 15 to 20 minutes, or until squash is tender when pierced with a fork.

Split Pea – Indian Dahl
Serves 6

1 large onion, chopped
1 small green pepper, chopped
1-1/2 cups yellow split peas
3 cups water
1/2 cup water
1-1/2 tsp black mustard seeds
1 tsp turmeric
1/2 tsp curry powder
1 lemon juiced

Simmer split peas in 3 cups water for 30 minutes or until tender. Add more water, if needed. In another saucepan, simmer chopped onions, green peppers, turmeric, curry powder, mustard seeds and 1/2 cup water for 15 minutes or until onions and peppers are tender. Mix with peas and add lemon juice. Serve over a generous portion of brown rice.

Stir Fry – Sesame Bok Choy & Carrot
Serves 2

5 cups bok choy, cut into 1/2-inch pieces
4 cloves garlic, minced
3 carrots, cut diagonally into 1/4-inch slices
3 cups cooked quinoa
1/2 cup chopped green onions
1/4 cup vegetable broth
2 tsp minced ginger root
2 tbsp toasted sesame seeds

In a large skillet or wok, stir-fry garlic, carrots and green onions in 3 tbsp vegetable broth for 3 minutes. Add bok choy and stir-fry another 2 minutes. Stir in vegetable broth and ginger. Reduce heat and simmer 5 minutes. Sprinkle sesame seeds over stir-fry. Spoon over quinoa.

Stir Fry – Vegetables
Makes 4 to 6 servings.

3 carrots, cut into 2-inch strips
2 green onions, chopped
1 medium onion, sliced
1 green pepper, sliced
2 cups cooked rice
1 cup cauliflower florets
1 cup broccoli florets
1 cup snow peas
1 cup sliced mushrooms
1/4 cup low-sodium Tamari (soy sauce)
1/4 cup lemon juice
1/3 cup vegetable broth
1-2 tsp grated fresh ginger root

Mix together the Tamari, lemon juice, and ginger. Heat the broth in a large pan and add the cauliflower, broccoli, carrots, onion, green pepper. Stir frequently, cooking evenly. Add the snow peas, mushrooms, and green onions. Continue to stir frequently until the vegetables are cooked but still crunchy. Serve over rice, topped with the marinade.

Tabouli
Serves 6

4 green onions, chopped
1 cucumber, chopped
1 tomato, chopped
1 red pepper, chopped
1 cup boiling water
1 cup bulgur
1/2 cup parsley, minced

Let soak for 30 minutes bulgur and boiling water or until water is absorbed: Stir in remaining ingredients. Toss well and chill. Add favorite dressing.

Tabouli – Quinoa
Serves 4 to 6

2 small tomatoes
3 green onions, chopped
2-1/2 cups cooked quinoa (1 cup dry)
2 cups finely chopped parsley
3/4 cup chopped mint
1/2 cup diced seedless cucumbers
3 tbsp lemon juice
1 tbsp vegetable broth
1/4 tsp black pepper

Rinse quinoa thoroughly. Bring 1 cup quinoa and 1-3/4 cup water to a full boil over medium heat, cover, and reduce to simmer. Continue simmering for 15 minutes. Remove from heat and uncover. Allow to cool. In a bowl, combine quinoa, mint, cucumbers, parsley, tomatoes, and onions. In a small bowl, whisk together the lemon juice, broth and pepper. Pour over salad; toss. Serve at room temperature or refrigerate and serve cold.

Tacos and More

Brown rice
Cooked black beans (*See Rules for Meal Preparation, Bean Preparation*)
Chopped tomatoes
Chopped videlia, green or any onion
Frozen corn thawed in hot water
Chopped red, yellow or green peppers
Grated or julienned carrots
Water chestnuts
Chopped cilantro
Chopped arugala
Low-sodium Tamari (soy sauce)
Salsa
Taco shells (whole wheat)

Cook rice. Heat beans. Put all chopped vegetables in individual dishes. Start on your plate with rice and just pile it up high and top it all with low-sodium Tamari and/or salsa. Put all leftovers in a bowl and use for salad the next day adding balsamic vinegar.

Vegetables – Grilled
Makes about 4 servings

2 ears fresh corn
1 red onion
1 red bell pepper
1 medium zucchini or other summer squash
2 cups button mushrooms
2 tsp vegetable broth
2 tsp garlic granules or powder
2 tsp mixed Italian herbs
2 tsp chili powder

Preheat grill. Cut onion, bell pepper, and zucchini into generous chunks. Place in a large mixing bowl. Clean mushrooms and add. Husk corn, cut it into 1-inch lengths, and add. Sprinkle vegetables with broth and toss to coat. Sprinkle with garlic granules, Italian herbs and chili powder. Toss to mix. Spread vegetables in a single layer on a grilling rack and place over medium-hot coals. Cover and cook 5 minutes. Turn with a spatula and cook until tender when pierced with a sharp knife, about 5 more minutes. Repeat with remaining vegetables.

Wrap – Quickie

Whole wheat wraps
Broccoli
Sliced beets
Radishes
Chopped tomatoes
Garlic clove
Romaine lettuce

You can make as many wraps from this as you want, depending on what you have in the refrigerator. Steam the broccoli lightly so it is still crisp. Put it at the base of the wrap, and then add all the other ingredients, with lettuce on top. Sprinkle with Tabasco, if desired.

Wrap – Thai Wraps
Serves 6

6 large tortillas
1 small onion, chopped
1 carrot, thinly sliced
1 celery stalk, thinly sliced
1/2 red bell pepper, diced
2 cups sliced mushrooms
2 cups finely chopped kale
2 cups cooked brown rice
1/2 cup chopped cilantro
6 tbsp Plum Sauce
1 tbsp peanut butter
2 tbsp low-sodium Tamari (soy sauce)
1-1/2 tsp curry powder

Mix the peanut butter with 3 tablespoons of water. Set aside. Heat 1/2 cup of water and the Tamari in a large skillet. Add the onion, carrot, celery, and mushrooms and cook until the vegetables are tender. Stir in the curry powder, red bell pepper, cilantro, kale, and peanut butter mixture. Cover and cook until the kale is tender. Heat the tortillas in a dry skillet until soft. Place about 1/2 cup of the vegetable mixture along the center of the tortilla. Top with 1/4 cup of brown rice and 2 tsp of Plum Sauce. Roll the tortilla around the filling.

Wrap – Veggie Wrap
Makes 4 wraps

4 large tortillas
1 carrot, shredded
1 cup bean sprouts
1–2 cups hummus
1–2 cups mixed salad greens or torn leaf lettuce
1/4 cup sunflower seeds

Preheat oven or toaster oven to 375. Place sunflower seeds in a small ovenproof dish and roast until lightly browned and fragrant. Set aside. Warm tortillas, one at a time, in a large dry skillet, flipping to warm both sides until soft and pliable. Spread each tortilla evenly with about 1/2 cup of hummus, leaving edges uncovered. Divide remaining ingredients evenly among tortillas. Wrap tortillas around filling.

Yams and Bok Choy
Serves 4

2 large cloves of garlic, minced
2 small bok choy, finely sliced
2 small yams, cut into bite-sized chunks
1 onion, sliced and quartered
1 tbsp vegetarian Worcestershire sauce
1/2 tsp Thai chili paste
1/2 lemon

Put yams in a deep skillet and just cover them with water. Cover skillet and boil yams 5 to 10 minutes until soft when pierced with a fork. Add onions and garlic and continue to simmer until about half of the water has boiled away. Add Worcestershire sauce, chili paste, and bok choy. Simmer until the bok choy is soft. Squeeze lemon over the mixture and serve.

Yams With Cranberries and Apples
Serves 8

4 yams, peeled
1 large, green apple, peeled and diced
1 cup raw cranberries
1/2 cup raisins
1/2 cup organic orange juice
2 tbsp maple syrup
Maple syrup

Preheat oven to 350. Cut peeled yams into 1-inch chunks and place in a large baking dish. Top with diced apple, cranberries, and raisins. Sprinkle with maple syrup or other sweetener, then pour orange juice over all. Cover and bake for 1 hour and 15 minutes, or until yams are tender when pierced with a fork.

Dips, Spreads and Sauces

Apple Chutney
Makes 3 cups

1-1/2 pounds tart apples (about 3 large apples)
1 medium garlic clove, minced
1 cup raw, maple syrup
1 cup cider vinegar
1/2 cup water
1 tbsp chopped fresh ginger or 1/2 tsp ground ginger
1 tsp each ground cinnamon and cloves
1/4 tsp cayenne, or more to taste

Coarsely chop the apples, then combine them with all the remaining ingredients in a heavy saucepan. Bring to a boil, then lower heat and simmer uncovered, stirring occasionally, for 1 hour, until most of the liquid is absorbed.

Bread Dressing
Makes about 4 cups

3 cups sliced mushrooms (about 1/2 pound)
2 celery stalks, thinly sliced
1 onion, chopped
4 cups cubed whole wheat bread
1 cup vegetable broth
1/3 cup finely chopped parsley
1 tbsp vegetable broth
1/2 tsp thyme
1/2 tsp marjoram
1/2 tsp sage
1/8 tsp black pepper

Sauté onion in broth until translucent. Add sliced mushrooms and celery. Cover and cook over medium heat, stirring occasionally, for 5 minutes. Preheat oven to 350. Stir bread into onion mixture, along with parsley, thyme, marjoram, sage, and black pepper. Lower heat and continue cooking 3 minutes, stirring often. Stir in vegetable broth, a little at a time, until dressing obtains desired moistness. Spread in a baking dish, cover and bake 20 minutes. Remove cover and bake 10 minutes longer.

Brown Gravy
Makes 2 cups

2 cups water or vegetable broth
3 tbsp low-sodium Tamari (soy sauce)
2 tbsp cornstarch
1 tbsp cashews
1 tbsp onion powder
1/2 tsp garlic granules or powder

Pour water or broth into a blender. Add cashews, onion powder, garlic granules, cornstarch, and Tamari. Blend until completely smooth, 2 to 3 minutes. Transfer to a saucepan and cook over medium heat, stirring constantly, until thickened.

"Cheese" Sauce

2 cups water
1/2 cup nutritional yeast flakes
1/2 cup whole wheat flour
1/2 tsp garlic powder
1/4 cup vegetable broth
1 tsp wet mustard

In a 2-quart saucepan, mix together nutritional yeast flakes, flour and garlic powder, then 2 cups water. Cook over medium heat, whisking until it thickens and bubbles. Cook 30 seconds more, then remove from head and whisk in vegetable broth and mustard. Sauce will thicken as it cools but will thin when heated. Good as a topping.

"Cheesy" Garbanzo Spread
Makes about 2 cups

2 cups dry garbanzo beans (*See Rules for Meal Preparation, Bean Preparation*)
1/2 cup roasted red peppers
3 tbsp vegetable broth
3 tbsp lemon juice

Place all ingredients in a food processor or blender. Process until very smooth. If using a blender, you will have to stop it occasionally and push everything down into the blades with a rubber spatula. The mixture should be quite thick, but to thin add a tablespoon of water.

Chunky Ratatouille Sauce
Serves 6

1 1/2 cups tomatoes, coarsely chopped
8 ounces of cremini mushrooms (also called baby bellas)
6 cloves garlic, minced
2 stalks celery, chopped
2 small onions, chopped
1 large eggplant, cut into 1-inch chunks
1/2 cup vegetable broth
1/4 to 1/2 cup water
1 tsp Italian herbs
1/2 tsp thyme
1/2 tsp black pepper (add more to taste)

Soak eggplant chunks in water for 10 minutes. Drain, rinse, and drain again. Braise onion, celery, and garlic in 1/4 cup of broth. When the vegetables are soft, add the eggplant chunks and 1/4 cup of water. Simmer, stirring occasionally, until the eggplant is soft. Add more water, if necessary, to keep mixture from drying out. Add mushrooms, spices, remaining wine, and tomatoes. Simmer for 5 minutes. Serve over whole wheat pasta shells, brown rice, or your favorite grain.

Cranberry Persimmon Relish
Makes about 2 cups

2 fuyu persimmons
1 cup cranberries, fresh or frozen
2 tbsp orange juice concentrate
1 tbsp maple syrup
1/2 tsp ginger

Remove stems, then coarsely chop persimmons in a food processor. Add cranberries, orange juice concentrate, syrup and ginger. Process using quick pulses until coarsely and uniformly chopped. Let stand 20 minutes before serving.

Garlic Bean Dip
Serves 2

2 cloves garlic, minced
1-1/2 tbsp vegetable broth
1/3 pound green beans
1 tsp low-sodium Tamari (soy sauce)
1/2 tsp onion powder

Steam green beans for 10 minutes in about a cup of water until tender. Rinse beans under cold water when done. Place remaining ingredients in a blender or food processor. Add cooked beans. Blend 2 minutes or until creamy. Serve with whole wheat crackers.

Guacamole
Serves 6

1 avocado
2 cups cooked peas or 1 cup cooked green beans
2 tbsp chopped onion
1/4 cup salsa (or more to taste)
2 tbsp fresh lime juice

Blend the avocado and peas or green beans together in a blender, until smooth. Stir in the onion and salsa. Just before serving, stir in the fresh lime juice.

Hummus Dip
Makes 2 cups

2 cups dry garbanzo beans (*See Rules for Meal Preparation, Bean Preparation*)
1 garlic clove (or more to taste)
2 (or more) tbsp of vegetable broth (add more if needed for consistency)
2 tbsp of lemon juice
1/4 tsp ground cumin.

Put everything in a food processor and let it rip until smooth.

Maple Sweet Potato Spread
Makes about 2 cups

3 dried figs, finely chopped
1 large sweet potato, peeled and quartered
1 small onion, peeled and quartered
1 tbsp water
1 tbsp maple syrup

Steam sweet potato and onion pieces until soft. Transfer to a food processor with remaining ingredients. Blend until thick and smooth. Pour into a small container. Keep covered and refrigerate until ready to serve.

Peanut Sauce
Serves 5 to 8

1 cup low-sodium Tamari (soy sauce)
1 cup peanut butter
1/4 cup water
1/4 cup cooking sherry
1 cup lemon or lime juice
2 tbsp minced fresh garlic
1 tbsp red curry paste
1/2 tbsp onion powder
1/2 tbsp basil
1/2 tsp cayenne
1/4 tsp paprika
2 to 3 dashes of Tabasco

Mix all ingredients using a whisk or blender, until creamy.

Plum Sauce

1 17-ounce can purple plums in heavy syrup
2 garlic cloves
2 tbsp seasoned rice vinegar
1 tbsp cornstarch
1 tbsp low-sodium Tamari (soy sauce)
1/8 tsp cayenne (more or less to taste)

Remove pits from the plums, then purée plums in a blender or food processor along with their liquid and the remaining ingredients. Heat in a saucepan, stirring constantly, until thickened.

Refried Beans
Makes about 5 cups

1 1/2 cups dry pinto beans
1 4-ounce can diced green chilies
4 garlic cloves, minced or pressed
1 onion, chopped
1 cup crushed or finely chopped tomatoes
1 1/2 tsp cumin
1/4 tsp cayenne

Clean and rinse beans, then soak in about 6 cups of water for 6 to 8 hours. Discard soaking water, rinse beans and place in a large pot with 4 cups of fresh water, minced garlic, cumin, and cayenne. Simmer until tender, about 1 hour. Heat 1/2 cup of water in a large skillet. Add onion and cook until soft, about 5 minutes. Stir in tomatoes and diced chilies. Cook, uncovered, over medium heat for 10 minutes, stirring occasionally. Add cooked beans, including some cooking liquid, a cup at a time to tomato mixture. Mash some of the beans as you add them. When all the beans have been added, stir to mix, then cook over low heat, stirring frequently, until thickened.

Salsa Fresca
Makes about 6 cups

1 1/2 cups tomato sauce
4 ripe tomatoes, chopped (about 4 cups)
4 garlic cloves, minced
1 small onion, finely chopped
1 bell pepper, finely chopped
1 jalapeño pepper, seeded and finely chopped or 1 teaspoon red pepper flakes
(more or less to taste)
1 cup chopped cilantro leaves
2 tbsp cider vinegar
1-1/2 tsp cumin

Combine all ingredients in a mixing bowl. Stir to mix. Let stand 1 hour before serving.

Desserts

Banana Cake
Serves 8

4 ripe bananas
2 cups whole wheat pastry flour
1-1/2 tsp baking soda
1 cup chopped walnuts
1/2 cup maple syrup (or to taste)
1/3 cup applesauce
1/4 cup water
1 tsp vanilla extract

Preheat oven to 350. Mix flour, baking soda in a bowl. In a large bowl, beat maple syrup, applesauce together. Add bananas and mash them. Stir in water and vanilla, mix thoroughly. Add flour mixture, chopped walnuts and stir to mix. Spread in a 9-inch square baking pan. Bake for 45 to 50 minutes, or until a toothpick inserted into the center comes out clean.

Berry Cobbler
One 9 x 9-inch cobbler

Berry mixture:
5-6 cups fresh or frozen berries (blueberries, blackberries, raspberries, or a mixture)
1/4 cup whole wheat pastry flour
1/2 cup natural sweetener

Topping:
1 cup whole wheat pastry flour
2/3 cup non-dairy milk
2 tbsp natural sweetener
1-1/2 tsp baking powder

Preheat oven to 375. Spread berries in a 9 x 9-inch baking dish. Mix in flour and sugar. Place in oven until hot or about 15 minutes. To prepare topping, mix flour, sugar, baking powder in a bowl. Add non-dairy milk and stir until batter is smooth. Spread evenly over hot berries, then bake until golden brown, 25 to 30 minutes.

Fruit Compote
Makes 2 cups

2 cups sliced fresh peaches
2 cups hulled fresh strawberries
1/2 cup white grape juice concentrate or apple juice concentrate

In a large saucepan combine all ingredients. Bring to a simmer and cook for about 5 minutes, or until fruit just becomes soft. Serve warm or cold.

Gingered Melon Wedges
Serves 6

1 large cantaloupe
1 tbsp natural sweetener
1 tbsp candied ginger (optional)
1/2 tsp ground ginger

Cut melon in half and seed. Then cut each half into chunks. Stir together sweetener and ground ginger. Sprinkle over melon chunks and chill.

Nutty Fruit Balls
Makes about 30 pieces

2/3 cup raisins
2/3 cup golden raisins
2/3 cup dried apricots
2/3 cup dried figs
2/3 cup cashews
1/2 cup peanut butter
1/2 cup carob powder
1/3 cup pitted dates

Grind the dried fruits and nuts into small pieces in a food grinder or heavy-duty food processor. Add the peanut butter and carob powder, mixing thoroughly. Roll into balls the size of walnuts.

Peaches (flambé) with Berries

Fresh or frozen raspberries or blueberries
1 ripe peach
 2 tsp natural sweetener
1 tsp lemon juice

Wash and halve peach. Remove pit. Place peach half, flat side up, in center of a square piece of doubled aluminum foil. Fill cavity of peach half with fresh or frozen raspberries or blueberries. Sprinkle the sweetener and lemon juice on the top. Wrap in foil. Grill approximately 15-20 minutes over hot flame, turning once.

Pudding – Brown Rice
Makes about 3 cups

2 cups cooked brown rice
1 1/2 cups water
1/3 cup raisins
1/4 cup maple syrup
1 tbsp cornstarch
1/4 tsp cinnamon
1 tsp vanilla

Whisk water and cornstarch together in a medium saucepan. Add cooked rice, maple syrup, raisins, and cinnamon. Simmer over medium heat 3 minutes, stirring constantly. Remove from heat and stir in vanilla. Serve warm or cold.

Pudding – Sweet Potato
Makes about 1 1/2 cups

1 cup cooked sweet potato or yam
1/2 cup water
1/3 cup rolled oats
1 tbsp maple syrup
1/4 tsp cinnamon

Combine all ingredients in a blender and blend until smooth.

Pudding – Rice
Makes 6 1/2-cup servings

2 cups cooked brown rice
1-1/2 cups water
3 tbsp raisins
2 tbsp maple syrup
1 tsp vanilla extract
1/4 tsp cinnamon
1/4 tsp vanilla extract

In a medium-size saucepan, combine all ingredients and bring to a slow simmer. Cook uncovered for about 20 minutes, or until thick. Serve hot or cold.

Pudding – Vanilla
Makes about 3 cups

2 cups water
1 cup cooked, peeled yam
5 tbsp maple syrup
2 tbsp cornstarch
1 tbsp potato flour
1/2 tsp vanilla extract

Combine water, cooked yam, and maple syrup in a blender and process until completely smooth. With blender running, add cornstarch, potato flour and vanilla extract. Transfer to a saucepan and heat, stirring constantly, until mixture bubbles and thickens. Remove from heat and transfer to individual serving dishes if desired. Cool before serving.

Rainbow Delight
Serves 6

2 apples, grated
2 carrots, grated
2/3 cup shredded coconut
1/2 cup raisins
1/2 cup chopped walnuts

Toss all ingredients together in a bowl and serve.

Recipes on the Web

The recipes contained in this book are meant to be only representative samples and a book cannot contain the wealth of possible meals that can be made with the RAVE Diet. To that end, there are thousands of recipes you can conveniently look up and search for on the Internet. Below are just a few of the web sites containing recipes for every occasion.

In many cases, you will have to make slight changes to these recipes so they conform to the RAVE rules (e.g., substitute white pasta with whole wheat pasta and use oil substitutes. See *Cooking Without Oil*.)

The best and most extensive recipe archive, in my opinion, is the first one, FatFree.com.

FatFree.com
www.fatfree.com/
Asian Recipes
www.asiarecipe.com/
Recipe Source
www.recipesource.com/special-diets/vegetarian/
The Vegan Chef
www.veganchef.com/
Vegetarians in Paradise
www.vegparadise.com/recipeindex.html
VegWeb Recipes
www.vegweb.com/food/

Food Lists

The following are lists of foods to provide you with suggestions and to also show you the wide variety of foods that available with the RAVE Diet.

Breads

(whole wheat only)

Bagel
Bread - Italian
Bread - French
Bread - pumpernickel
Bread - whole wheat
Bread - rye - American - light
Bread - mixed whole grain
Bread - pita

Bread - oatmeal and bran
Corn taco shells - organic
Muffin - English
Roll - homemade
Spelt and sprouted grain breads
Sprouted whole wheat

Fruits

Apple
Apricot
Avocado
Bananas
Blackberries
Blueberries
Boysenberries
Breadfruit
Carambola
Carissa
Cherimoya
Cherries
Cranberries
Dates
Elderberries
Figs
Gooseberries
Grapefruit
Grapes
Guavas

Kiwifruit
Lemons
Limes
Loganberries
Longans
Loquats
Lychees
Mangos
Melons - cantaloupe
Melons - casaba
Melons - honeydew
Mulberries
Nectarines
Oranges
Papayas
Passion fruit
Peaches
Pears
Persimmons
Pineapple

Pitanga
Plantains
Plums
Pomegranates
Pricklypears
Prunes
Pummelo
Quinces
Raisins
Raspberries
Roselle
Sapodilla
Sapotes
Soursop
Strawberries
Tamarinds
Tangerines
Watermelon

Nuts and Seeds

For nuts, get raw only

Almonds
Beech
Brazil
Breadfruit
Cashews
Chestnuts
Coconut
Filbert/hazel
Hickory
Macadamia
Peanut butter – (make your own)

Peanuts
Pecans
Pine nuts
Pistachio
Pumpkin/squash seeds
Sesame seeds
Soybean kernels
Sunflower seeds
Walnut
Walnuts

Pasta

Brown rice pasta
Organic soy pasta
Spelt pasta

Lentil pasta
Quinoa pasta
Whole wheat pasta

Vegetables

Alfalfa seeds - sprouted
Amaranth
Artichokes
Asparagus
Balsam pear
Bamboo shoots
Beans - Great Northern
Beans - green
Beans - snap - yellow/wax
Beans - black
Beans - French
Beans - adzuki
Beans - garbanzo
Beans - green
Beans - lima
Beans - mung
Beans - navy
Beans - red kidney beans
Beans - small white
Beets
Beet greens

Broccoli
Brussels sprouts
Burdock root
Cabbage - savoy
Cabbage - celery
Cabbage - common
Cabbage - red
Cabbage - white mustard
Carrot
Cauliflower
Celery - pascal
Chard - Swiss
Chicory greens
Chickpeas
Chinese vegetables mixed
Chives
Collards
Corn
Cress
Cucumber
Dandelion greens

Eggplant
Endive
Escarole
Fennel
Garlic
Ginger root
Gourd - white flowered
Hummus
Jerusalem artichokes
Kale
Kohlrabi
Leeks
Lentils
Lettuce - red leaf
Lettuce - romaine
Lettuce – butter head
Lotus root
Miso - fermented soybeans
Mung bean sprouts
Mushrooms
Mustard greens
Natto - fermented soybeans
Chestchinese
Okra
Onions - mature
Onions - young green
Parsley
Parsnips
Peas - edible podded
Peas - blackeye/cowpeas

Peas - snow pea pods
Peas – split green
Peppers - sweet
Peppers - hot chili
Poi - taro root product
Potato - baked - whole
Potato skin - baked
Pumpkin
Radishes
Rutabaga
Seaweed - spirulina
Seaweed - kelp (kombu)
Shallots
Soybeans - sprouted
Soybeans - green
Spinach
Squash - acorn
Squash - zucchini
Squash - butternut
Squash - summer
Sweet potato
Taro leaf
Taro root
Tomatoes
Turnip greens
Turnips
Water chestnuts
Watercress
Yam - mountain - Hawaii
Zucchini

Whole Grains

Amaranth
Pearled barley
Barley flakes
Basmati rice (brown)
Buckwheat
Bulgur
Couscous
Cornmeal
Cracked wheat
Kamut – whole grain

Kamut flakes
Matzos
Matzo meal
Millet
Popcorn – air popped
Quinoa
Rice - brown
Rolled oats
Rye
Spelt

Spelt flakes
Steel cut oats
Teff
Wehani rice
Wheat, cracked
Wheat flakes
Wheat germ
Wild rice

Recipe Index

General Index

Herceptin, 13, 39
high-protein, 139, 140
hormonal cancers, 68, 92
hormone, 141
hormones, 59, 60, 63, 68, 69, 70, 71, 84, 112, 114, 144
Humphrey, Hubert, 25, 26
hydrogenated oils, 97, 166
IGF-1, 92
immune system, 3, 4, 7, 26, 28, 32, 36, 38, 40, 49, 51, 52, 56, 57, 59, 60, 61, 62, 66, 70, 71, 73, 75, 76, 88, 89, 90, 96, 98, 103, 111, 124, 132, 134, 160, 162
insulin, 59, 82, 92, 138, 144
Interleukin II, 76
Jones, Hardin, 11, 40, 43
Kellogg, Harvey, 73
Kushi Institute, 21, 59
laetrile, 121, 126, 127
Leakey, Richard, 64
Lourdes, 75
macrobiotic, 79, 117
mammography, 5, 15, 28, 29, 30, 31, 32, 33, 34, 35, 36
mastectomy, 24, 31, 33, 111
McDonald's, 62
McDougall, John, 4, 15, 30, 50, 64, 98, 100, 139, 141
Mediterranean diet, 99
menopause, 141
mercury, 71, 84, 90, 95
metabolism, 58, 63, 86, 90, 103, 104, 135, 139
metastasis, 16, 19, 21, 24, 25, 27, 30, 31, 32, 38, 40, 43, 48, 60, 61, 67, 69, 95, 96, 98, 219, 245, 249
micronutrients, 6, 7, 56, 57, 61, 82, 84, 85, 93, 106, 110, 118, 120, 121, 146, 147, 160
Moss, Ralph, 17, 18, 21, 22, 24, 27, 37, 46, 126, 127
mother's milk, 72, 134, 140, 143
mucoid plaque, 74

National Breast Cancer Awareness Month, 45
National Cancer Institute, 9, 18, 19, 28, 31, 33, 34, 35, 37, 44, 46, 129, 138, 144
National Institutes of Health, 21
needle biopsy, 40
Newtonian view, 47
nocebo, 2
oil substitutes, 109, 149, 271
Okinawans, 128
olive oil, 97, 98, 99, 100
Omega-3's, 60, 98, 108
oncogene AC, 32
organochlorides, 45
organophosphate, 132
Ornish, Dean, 20, 97, 100, 129
osteoporosis, 45, 125, 134, 139, 140, 141, 142, 143
oxygen, 3, 63, 65, 70, 97, 102, 103, 116, 140, 160
oxygen, low, 65
pancreatic enzymes, 89
paraquat, 132
Parkinson's disease, 79, 132
Pasteur, Louis, 61
PCB's, 72, 95
pesticides, 69, 71, 72, 73, 106, 131, 132, 144, 147, 167, 168
phytochemicals, 49, 56, 80, 96, 106
placebo, 2, 11, 12, 16, 22, 76, 120, 122
prescription drugs, 26, 71, 72
Presley, Elvis, 74
Pritikin, Nathan, 49, 96, 141
protein, 139, 140, 142
protein, high, 63, 80, 113, 133, 134, 138, 139
protein, low, 63, 87
radiation
    causing breast cancer, 31, 33
    cumulative exposure, 35
relative numbers, 13, 14, 15, 29, 30
response rates, 22, 26

rule breakers, 7, 8
saturated fat, 94, 143
scurvy, 51, 121
Siegel, Bernie, 2, 8, 76
Sloan-Kettering Cancer Center, 45, 126, 127
Snow, Tony, 26
Sorafenib, 13
spontaneous regressions, 33, 55
superfood, 79, 80
supplements, 6, 7, 79, 84, 107, 118, 119, 120, 121, 123, 125, 126, 142
Tamoxifen, 13, 15, 19, 20, 45
terminal patients, 17, 21, 59, 111, 117, 122, 125
testosterone, 69, 70

Thermography, 36
true positive, 34
tumor shrinkage, 22, 25, 26, 27
U.S. Preventive Services Task Force, 38
Ulrich, Abel, 42, 120
untreated patients, 34, 40
vegetable oils, 60, 96, 97, 98, 99, 100, 101, 166
visceral fat, 59
vitamin C, 51, 118, 121, 125, 126
vitamin D, 79, 92, 103, 108, 123, 124, 125, 141, 142
Warburg, Otto, 65
Wayne, John, 74
WHEL Study, 49

References

For other books, articles and references beyond those cited in the footnotes, please visit www.RaveDiet.com.